# VAGUS NERVE: ACCESS YOUR BODY'S NATURAL HEALING POWER!

*Self Help Techniques and Exercises to Activate Your Vagus Nerve Stimulation, Overcoming Anxiety, Autism, Inflammation, Trauma, Depression, Chronic Illness and more.*

**Stephen W. Rosenberg and Emeran M. Navaz**

Vagus Nerve: Access Your Body's Healing Power! Copyright © 2019 by Stephen W. Rosenberg and Emeran M. Navaz. All Rights Reserved.

All rights reserved. No part of this book may be reproduced in any form or by any electronic or mechanical means including information storage and retrieval systems, without permission in writing from the author. The only exception is by a reviewer, who may quote short excerpts in a review.

# CONTENTS

PART ONE .................................................................. 1

Chapter 1: Vagus Nerve ............................................. 3

Chapter 2: Polyvagal Theory ..................................... 11

Chapter 3: Human Emotions ..................................... 19

PART TWO ................................................................ 33

Chapter 1: Trauma .................................................... 35

Chapter 2: Polyvagal Theory and Trauma ................. 39

Chapter 3: De-activating ........................................... 54

Chapter 4: Window of Tolerance .............................. 59

Chapter 5: Co-Regulating ......................................... 71

Chapter 6: Stories We Tell Ourselves ....................... 91

Chapter 7: Somatic Experiencing .................................................. 99

Chapter 8: Play In A Polyvagal World ................................. 103

Chapter 9: Music ...................................................... 109

Chapter 10: Social Media .......................................... 113

Chapter 11: Create Safety .......................................... 117

PART THREE ...................................................... 121

Chapter 1: Polyvagal and Autism ........................................ 123

Chapter 2: Cognitive Behavioral Therapy ........................... 133

Chapter 3: Guided Imagery ................................................... 137

PART FOUR ...................................................... 141

Chapter 1: Vagus Nerve and the Body ................................. 143

Chapter 2: Toning Your Vagus ............................................. 153

Chapter 3: Better Breathing ................................................. 165

Conclusion ............................................................................. 171

Questions for further study ................................................. 173

REFERENCES ....................................................................... 177

# PART ONE

We often live with deep physical and emotional pain that lasts for days, months, even years. What if there were a simple solution that could help relieve much of life's pain, both the physical sort and the emotional sort?

Perhaps you have come looking for relief from stress or anxiety. Perhaps you suffer with depression, or epilepsy. Perhaps you have a deep emotional trauma that has left you scarred and reaching for help anywhere you can find it.

Perhaps your physical pains involve arthritis or chronic migraine. Perhaps you deal with digestive issues and neck pain. We will be looking at the body's superpower, the vagus nerve, its impact on every system in the body, and how toning it and keeping it healthy can bring relief for some of our most insidious, incurable, and painful maladies. The more scientists have learned about the function of this nerve bundle, the more excited the world has become over its potential use in treating a multitude of conditions, both minor illnesses and serious chronic, even debilitating conditions.

Its impact cannot be overstated.

We will take an in-depth look at the Polyvagal Theory as proposed by Professor Stephen Porges, Ph.D., and discuss its impact on how we interact with the world around us, how we respond to danger and feelings of safety, and how that can work together to bring healing in many ways.

Join us as we explore the Polyvagal Theory and how you can begin your journey to healing.

# CHAPTER 1: VAGUS NERVE

## Introducing the Nerve

First we are going to start with a little bit of science, then some explanation for people who are not research scientists or brain surgeons. We will be delving into some examples, both imaginary and personal stories that happened to real people. But first, we need to explore exactly what the vagus nerve is and how it interacts with the rest of the body in order to fully comprehend its impact on so many different areas of our lives.

The vagus nerve is the longest cranial nerve in the body, reaching out from the brain stem as a pair of nerves, one for controlling each side of the body. It got its name from the Latin word for *wanderer (vagus)* because it wanders throughout the entire body. This is an apt description as the vagus nerve impacts in some way nearly every organ in the body.

The vagus nerve prevents inflammation, acts as a conduit for information from the visceral lower abdominal organs to the brain, controls breathing, strengthens memory power, controls heart rate, and relays information from the facial muscles to the brain stem. The vagus nerve even has a connection to our taste buds.

Additionally, the vagus nerve impacts our creativity, our higher cognitive functions, and decision making.

Acting as the balance to the sympathetic nervous system, it helps to calm you when you are stressed, sending out signals to all the organs to release calming enzymes and proteins, thus providing the balance for the body's autonomic fight, flight, or freeze response, and stress levels.

# Form and Function of the Vagus Nerve

The human body has twelve cranial nerves that extend directly from the brain and brain stem, unlike spinal nerves that attach directly to the spinal cord. These cranial nerves act as information pathways from all the various parts of the body to the brain.

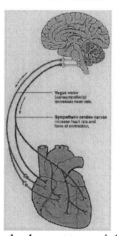

The vagus nerve is the longest cranial nerve, leading from the brain, along the jawline and extending down between the internal jugular vein and the internal carotid artery, through the neck and chest, into the abdomen and reaching down to the viscera, or intestines. This nerve mostly works to bring information from the organs to the central nervous system, so most of its information is going from the organs to the brain.

The vagus nerve is actually a bundle of two, the ventral and the dorsal. The ventral vagus extends from the right side to the heart and lungs impacting both heart rate and respirations, and into the facial muscles, eyes, and into the inner ear. You might notice that these are all parts of our body that deal with social engagement. This will be important later on. This part of the vagus nerve is myelinated. Myelin is a fatty substance that surrounds our nerve cell axons. It insulates them and acts as a means of speeding up the process by which those axons carry information. The greater the amount of myelinization present, the faster the speed of the information being carried to and from the brain.

The dorsal vagus extends from the left down into the abdomen and the lower organs, the guts. It is this part of the vagus that you are referring to when you say you have "a gut feeling" or someone "gets on your last nerve." This portion of the vagus nerve has no myelin.

All these descriptions give the sense that the vagus nerve is just one long line, but in fact it is a branching system that reaches into every part of your body like a tree root in soil, as the picture shows.

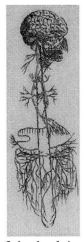

The vagus nerve is part of the body's parasympathetic nervous system. The sympathetic nervous system is what kicks in when you are in danger. It provides you with the fight or flight instinct when presented with some sort of sudden, unexpected, or threatening situation.

As part of the parasympathetic portion of the autonomic nervous system, the vagus nerve acts as an inhibitor for the sympathetic system, providing a counterbalance to the initial panic from the sympathetic system, and allowing the body to calm down.

The vagus nerve's motor functions extend to the medulla oblongata - where autonomic responses are regulated by the brain, while its sensory functions are directly tied to the cranial neural crest, where the body's facial muscles reside. This means the vagus nerve is informed and impacted by the very gestures of our face. We teach our own bodies how we feel based on how we are reacting to the world around us.

The vagus nerve is connected to the neuroception system of the body which helps us gather information to determine the safety of our environment on an unconscious level.

Another aspect of the vagus nerve is that fully 80% of all the information is traveling from the organ systems up this nerve to the brain, while only the remaining 20% of its function involves information traveling down the nerve to the organs and lower systems. We usually think of the brain as being the originator of all information regarding our surroundings, but really it is the individual systems that begin the process, such as the eyes that see telling us what our surroundings look like, ears that hear telling us what sounds are nearby, the nose gathering in and reacting to scents constantly, and the taste buds on the tongue telling us what we need to know about the food we put in our mouth. Skin receptors tell us what the air feels like, what we are touching at the time, and many other things that we only pick up on a subconscious level.

## Physical Damage to the Vagus Nerve

Physically, the vagus nerve can be damaged, of course.

The vagus nerve can be damaged by diabetes, upper respiratory viral infections, alcoholism, or through an accident during an operation. Stress, fatigue, anxiety, and even bad posture can also have a negative impact on the vagus nerve.

The symptoms of vagal nerve damage include loss of the gag reflex, difficulty speaking or complete loss of voice, a speaking voice that is hoarse or wheezy, trouble drinking liquids, unusual heart rate, abnormal blood pressure, pain in the ear, decreased production of stomach acid, nausea or vomiting, and abdominal bloating or pain. The health of the vagus nerve can be checked by testing the heart variability rate, the difference in heart rate between exhalation and inhalation. A steady, smooth rate indicates the health of the vagus nerve.

# CHAPTER 2: POLYVAGAL THEORY

## Polyvagal Theory

The polyvagal theory was first developed in 1994 by Professor Stephen Porges, Ph.D., director of the Brain-Body Center at the University of Chicago in Illinois. In this theory, Dr. Porges proposed a new way of dealing with how our body automatically reacts to intense challenges and situations.

Polyvagal refers to the dual systems that comprise the vagus nerve, ventral and dorsal, and how bringing that nerve into a place of safety greatly heightens the efficacy of basic social interactions, medical procedures, and even mental and emotional therapy.

Dr. Porges calls it triggering a feeling of safety, and so allowing the autonomic nervous system to help with the restoration of health in the body.

Dr. Porges proposed that while researchers understood the nervous system to be comprised of a sympathetic system and a parasympathetic system, he suggests that our bodies also have a third system that had been largely ignored beforehand, that of a neurologically based system of social engagement.

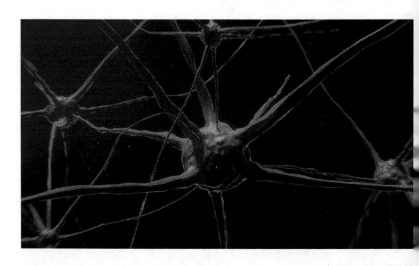

The vagus nerve has essentially two pathways, dorsal and ventral. These two pathways are said to have developed at different times through the evolutionary process of the human body, with the dorsal pathway being first, or oldest. This is the pathway that gives us our primal instincts for survival and preservation of life. Afterward, the ventral path functions then developed, receiving information from our facial muscles, eyes and ears, and observation of body language. This allows humans to have complex social interactions, such as collaboration and close relationships, based on the information we get from the outward bodily cues of others, as well. The newer system is able to inhibit the older ones, giving us control over our more primitive instincts. It is when these newer systems break down or prove inadequate that our older ones take over.

## Polyvagal Theory Explained

The polyvagal theory suggests that the human body is designed to function best when in a state of safety. When at rest, cells can be restored, the mind and brain can reset, muscles are repaired, heart rate is regulated, and digestion can occur. Who does not want to be able to digest their food? This is the optimal state for a human body to be in.

Conversely, when in a state of danger, muscles are taut and ready for action, heart rate increases, adrenaline floods the body. Everything is focused on one thing - determining the body's necessary response to the danger present. In this state, the body is being controlled by the dorsal vagal system and is primed for either fight or flight.

The parasympathetic vagus nerve is also responsible for the third response to danger, the shutdown in all its various forms and degrees.

When the body is in a state of safety, mentally and physically, it is being controlled by the ventral vagal state, allowing the person to engage in social activities. In this state, the body is more receptive to touch, is relaxed and able to remain calm, can carry on conversations and collaborate with others. In the ventral state, we can use facial expressions and accurately interpret the facial expressions of others around us. Our heart rate slows, and our blood pressure decreases while our hormones remain balanced. We can filter other sounds out in order to focus fully on human voices instead. In the ventral state, we welcome physical closeness and emotional connection. It is a state of balance and calm, able to recognize cues of danger and yet still remain in control of our actions.

For instance, a person in a ventral state may know he is lost in a mall but can remain calm while still reacting appropriately to solving the problem he finds himself in. He can walk calmly along, perhaps even smile at a passerby or two, while looking for the door he came into to enter the mall in the first place. He may even be able to stop at the food court on his way out and enjoy a meal. On the other hand, a person in a dorsal vagal state who finds themselves lost in the mall, instead of remaining calm, may go running through the passageways, dragging his child behind him, shopping bags flailing and coat bouncing madly off his shoulder as he frantically tries to find a door that leads to the proper parking lot. He may even run from a security guard that is only trying to help, misinterpreting his approach as an aggressive posture.

A person in a dorsal vagal state may begin to lose control of his emotions, interpreting a multitude of things around him as threatening. He may begin to see expressions of worry and mistake them for anger. He may interpret the actions of a person who is reaching out to him physically in an attempt to help as an attempt at assault instead. It is common for those in a dorsal state to mistake neutral facial expressions as anger, for example.

As the vagus nerve regulates facial expression and responsive body language, the theory is that this nerve has a direct impact on social connection, and co-regulating - the ability to help each other come back to a feeling of safety.

When this co-regulating is interrupted, threatened, or abused, then the person is in danger of no longer having the correct social cues in place for proper self-regulation. If a person cannot recognize who is safe for them to engage with, then they may enter a state of instability or isolate themselves altogether, and the cycle continues.

In the polyvagal theory of neurology and therapy, everything we experience as humans will be impacted by whether or not we experience it through a state of safety or a state of danger. Therapy, medical procedures, social interactions will all be improved by experiencing them from a state of safety.

# CHAPTER 3: HUMAN EMOTIONS

## Biology of Human Emotions

Humans like to think of ourselves as complex creatures, filled with mystery and wonder. We insist on seeing our emotions as untamable, unknowable, and unpredictable like something magical that cannot be defined. But in fact, our emotions have a neurological, biological foundation. Does this make them any less real? No. They are no less real, but they are controllable. If they are biological, then we have power over them. We can be in charge.

Humans are designed to need each other. Our emotions bind us together, urge us to rely on those around us, push us to protect our family and rise above to greater challenges. At their foundations, those emotions provide a response to the environment around us and form a basis for a social structure that helps us navigate life together in the healthiest way possible. It is important then to understand how emotions tie into the body neurologically. By understanding this biological and neurological component, we can take charge of our body once again, making it work for us and not against us.

In the human body, the nervous system has three responses to danger - fight, flight, or freeze. The sympathetic system regulates the first two, fight or flight. If we encounter a threat that seems to be something we can overcome, we fight.

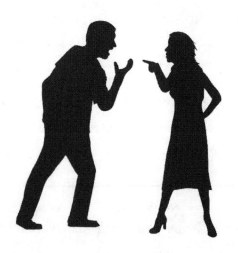

If the threat seems to be something we can escape from, we flee. But if the threat is both too powerful for us to fight and too swift for us to flee from it, then the parasympathetic system kicks back in again, causing a shutdown, usually partial in humans, but a freeze of some degree. These threats can be either physical or emotional, so that as humans we respond to emotional threats in these same stages as we do a physical threat to our life.

This third function of the parasympathetic system, the freeze, shutdown, or immobilization portion, is what allows us to fall asleep as well, so it is not always a negative thing. This immobilization allows us to remain calm when held in the arms of a trusted loved one or sit still and listen to the music of a babbling brook on a nature walk. This is what allows us to go into deep meditation or find that peaceful center of our own mind when in deep concentration. However, these positive aspects of immobilization do not occur when fear is also present. When immobilization occurs in humans while accompanied by fear it can and does cause deep trauma.

Think of the immobilization you may have witnessed in the animal kingdom. When a mother cat lifts her kitten by the nape of its neck, the kitten automatically goes limp. The kitten is not being harmed, but it goes into a state of immobilization during this process. On the other hand, when a wild animal is met with a threat such as a deer being chased down and caught by a lion, the deer will go through a period of shut down. If that shut down results in the lion becoming distracted, the deer can shift immediately back into flight mode and run away.

A wild animal can shift quickly back into flight, then join its herd and be back in its normal social state almost immediately. There is no great transition time needed. But with humans, this is not the case. A human forced into immobilization through fear will suffer some sort of trauma and will require help in some way to return back to a safe and social state of mind.

※ ※ ※

The polyvagal theory proposes that humans have a social engagement system based on the neurology of the vagus nerve system, and that it acts upon the lower systems - sympathetic and parasympathetic - to provide a counterbalance when we need to overcome those instincts to fight, flee, or freeze. This social engagement system gets its information from the facial muscles connected to the ventral portion of the vagus nerve, which is why being in a *safe and social state* is referred to as a *ventral state*.

Part of the polyvagal theory includes what is called a *vagal ladder*, describing the sympathetic response to a trauma, either a physical danger or an emotional one. The top of the ladder is the ventral state, where the person feels safe and has social connection with the people around him. In this state, heart rate is optimal, thinking and creativity are free to roam, blood pressure is stable, and digestion is promoted.

The next step down is the fight response, and immediately below that is flight. During these stages, digestion is slowed, heart rate increases, blood pressure goes up. Muscles are keyed for optimal movement, and higher thought processes are pushed to the side. For the moment when danger threatens, this is fine, but this is not a healthy state to live in long term.

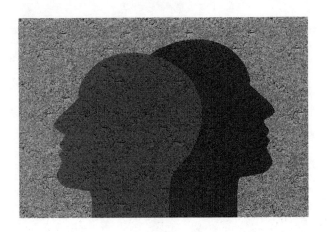

At the bottom is the dissociative state of freezing in place, a complete shut-down. When described as the bottom rung of this ladder, it is referring to the sort of immobilization, or shut down, that is accompanied by fear, and that is not a good thing for humans to experience.

You might see the fight or flight state referred to as the *sympathetic state* as well, and the freeze as a *dorsal state*. It is called dorsal because the dorsal portion of the vagus nerve ends in the lower abdomen and is the basest, last ditch effort stage of self-preservation.

These responses are also autonomic. This means they are an unconscious response to the cues the body is interpreting from the environment, and the signals being received from the body by the vagus nerve. When a person switches from the social and safe state down to a fight or flight state, it is an unconscious movement, one which they cannot easily control. Our body reacts, though once we have recognized what those reactions mean, we can then regain control.

The first rung of the vagal ladder as described above is safety and social connection. In this state, the person is able to function in all the normal areas of life. This is the ideal state to live in, one in which calm is in charge. Happiness and normal curiosity about life can occur, as well as healthy social connections, a robust immune system, lowered heart rate and blood pressure, and healthy digestion. All of this is automatically brought on by being in a ventral vagal state of calm. In this state, all the neurons are firing properly, we can interpret facial expressions and physical gestures from others accurately, and our stories regarding life around us are basically accurate.

When something comes along to threaten the safety of this environment, then the sympathetic nervous system kicks us out of the ventral state and into the next rung down on that vagal ladder. The nerves used to detect threats can gather information from sources we are not even consciously aware of, so at times we might be thrown into this state without fully understanding why.

In this state, the desire to stay alive is prime, and when threatened, the control shifts to the second state - that of threat assessment and protection. It is a base instinct that takes pre-eminence. Our body cares more about staying alive than it does about the ability to cognitively think about staying alive. Heart rates are raised, digestion slows, facial expressions are minimized, senses are focused on identifying threats, muscles tensed in preparation for fighting or fleeing.

This is why a drowning victim may fight his rescuer. He is responding to the threat against his life and so has been rendered incapable of rational thought. At that point, he is unable to calm himself and consider his environment, taking stock of what around him may or may not be a threat. Fight-or-flight has taken hold, and he is completely taken over by that reaction.

Some are living in a constant state of fight or flight. Gang members who live always on the alert for danger around them. A child living in an abusive home, even military troops deployed to the front lines of a combat zone.

Someone in this constant state of fight or flight can much more easily slide into the lowest and final stage, the freeze. Some call it dissociative, going limp, shutting down either emotionally or physically, sometimes both depending on where the threat is originating. This is again an unconscious reaction, not something the person is controlling voluntarily. A victim of a life-threatening or emotionally traumatic situation may freeze and then feel guilty for freezing.

Remember, this is a perfectly normal part of the self-preservation built into our neurological system. Freezing does not mean the person is inadequate or abnormal. It in fact means the nervous system is acting correctly, doing what it needed to do to try to preserve his life. The term freeze may also be inadequate to fully describe this state. There are various degrees of shut down, based on the individual. Literally freezing in place may not happen, but some level of emotional or psychological shut down may very well be occurring.

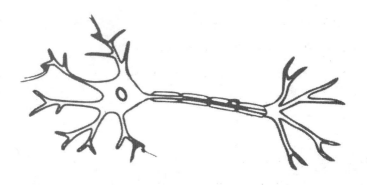

Historically speaking, the world has not been kind to the shut down state. We reward behavior that fights off a threat, and we empathize with behavior that runs from an overwhelming foe. But we have more typically seen the shut down mode as weakness, blaming ourselves for freezing, even considering it cowardice or somehow a sign of uncaring.

In one interview, Dr. Porges sums it up this way: *"The root of the Polyvagal Theory is the recognition that in the absence of the ability to fight or flee, the body's only effective defense is to immobilize and shut down."*

I heard of a case where two children were racing in a backyard while a third child watched nearby. Suddenly the racers changed course and ran to the back door intending to race inside. They did not know the sliding glass door had been shut, and they both ran straight into it, shattering the glass. This was before the current requirement of safety glass in doors like this, and there were injuries involved in accidents like this. The child behind the racers watching, instead of helping, went straight into a frozen state, the adults around wondering absently what was wrong with her. One was even quite angry with the child for not helping out, although that child had completely shut down neurologically and no longer had control of their own body.

What the adults did not realize was that this third child lived in a state of fight or flight at home, so a trauma like this sent her straight into a dissociative state. She was not trying to be unhelpful to the children who were hurt in the process of this accident. Rather the third child was in a state of shock, later recounting that she barely remembered anything surrounding that traumatic incident that night, her brain having almost completely shut down at the time. But because she was not physically harmed, her state of shock was not recognized by the adults.

While not physically in as much real danger as the ones who broke the glass, the response of the third child was just as much an autonomic response of her nervous system to dissociate from the situation in front of her. It was a self-preservation response just the same, and the child who experienced it should not carry the weight of guilt because of having gone through it.

Victims of emotional trauma often do not hear this. They feel great shame because they did not fight back or run away. Sometimes people will even ask them why they froze, why they did not fight back. What others do not realize, and often what the victim does not realize either, is that this freezing reaction-warrior is as much a part of the body's defense mechanism as the other two warriors are. The freeze, the immobilization, is neurological, and while fear-based immobilization is traumatic, it is also a natural thing.

Next, we will start to explore the ways the polyvagal theory can help us overcome emotional trauma.

# PART TWO

In the next section we will be taking a close look at trauma, the different types of traumas, how they affect us physiologically and mentally, and how the polyvagal theory is being used to help people on the journey of healing from these traumas.

# CHAPTER 1: TRAUMA

## Defined

What is trauma? The term is rather loosely defined and is generally talked about in terms of both emotional and psychological trauma. Psychological trauma focuses on the health of the mind, while emotional trauma revolves more around feelings.

Trauma is more than just stress. Our bodies return to normal functioning after a day or two when we experience a stressful moment or event. In cases where the person has been traumatized, their body does not return to that normal state. Scientists have even found through brain scans that our brains are changed when we are experiencing something traumatizing.

There is a biological component to trauma, changing us physically on the inside. This has been clearly shown through MRIs of brains before and after a traumatic event.

It is important to distinguish between average, manageable stress versus real trauma. We can tell the difference by how quickly we return to normal after the event.

Is the traumatic event still affecting your everyday life? Are you upset faster or more often? Are your reactions appropriate to the actual situation affecting you right then? Are you upset an extraordinary length of time? Do you have difficulty coming back to a calm state? Do you have flashbacks of the event that are startlingly realistic? Do you feel burdened or chained by these thoughts?

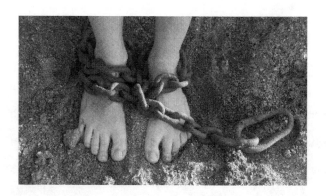

Even if we do not realize it, we can be experiencing trauma. It has sometimes been described as frozen in an active state of emotional intensity. No matter what causes it, emotional trauma happens when you experience something you were not expecting, were not prepared for, and had no way of preventing it. You were trapped in that event, and it overwhelmed you.

Psychological trauma involves more of an actual physical event, going through a natural disaster perhaps, or an assault or accident. Even a sports injury, when unexpected and devastating, can cause psychological trauma.

Any number of things can cause either psychological or emotional trauma. There are certain symptoms you can look out for if you think you have been traumatized. A few of them are:

- Eating or sleep disturbances
- Chronic unexplained pain
- Depression or anxiety
- Emotional numbness
- Withdrawal from family relationships
- Inability to concentrate

- Feeling distracted

This is by no means an exhaustive list. If you believe you might be experiencing the symptoms of trauma, please get help. Perhaps the next few chapters of this book will help you start your journey back to a place of health.

# CHAPTER 2: POLYVAGAL THEORY AND TRAUMA

## What is Trauma?

The polyvagal theory has had a profound impact on how we treat emotional trauma, as well as many psychosomatic disorders where physical symptoms arise from emotional or mental factors. In the past, much of the theory of therapy dealt with specific events, figuring out what had happened in the patient's past and how to deal with those issues. While I am not here to argue with that model of therapy, and this book is not about therapeutic practices in the professional field, the polyvagal theory approaches patient therapy in a slightly different way.

Using the polyvagal theory, you could think of your nervous system as employing three very different warriors in your body's defense.

The first is the Viking warrior, the fighter. He slashes and burns without thinking, going for the most effective route through any barrier that presents itself. This warrior is bold and brash and is thinking only about defense.

The second is Flash, the comic book superhero. His greatest superpower is running lightning fast and for a long time until the danger is far behind. He is thinking of only one thing - the swiftest, straightest path to getting away. Far away.

The third is a ninja. Stealth is key to this warrior. His defense is most often to lie in the shadows, to wait unseen, to immobilize until the danger has passed by. He is entirely consumed with remaining in the shadows.

Each of these warriors usually fights alone. Although the first two will sometimes blend a bit, working in conjunction with one another as if they were on the same wavelength, the ninja only works alone.

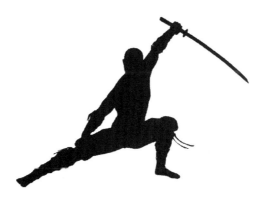

These warriors are meant to be temporary rules of our body, but trauma takes these three warriors and sets them in charge of the body full time. Instead of being hired for a temporary job, they unpack, settle in, and make themselves at home and in charge for the long haul. They become the masters instead of the servants.

Next, we will be talking about how these warriors accomplish the takeover – what gives them the power to remain in charge? And how can we take that power back?

# When Neuroception Goes Wrong

What counts to humans as a state of danger? What do we see as dangerous? This seems like a straightforward question with a very simple answer, but in reality, it is not. There are some things that are instantly and universally recognizable as a danger. For instance, we would see a lion prowling around our backyard as a dangerous situation and depending on our confidence level, we would either fight the lion or flee from it. We would see an approaching tornado as a dangerous situation, and we would instinctively flee.

There is another world of sensory input though, one called *neuroception*. Neuroception is the automatic detection of a threat as sensed by the automatic nervous systems in our bodies. We interpret tiny things around us and incorporate them into our overall sense of safety, whether we realize we are doing it or not. If a person is lower on the vagal ladder, they may interpret neutral faces as angry, for example. This is because our nervous system is always vigilant for threats, and if it is already in a hypervigilant state, then it is going to interpret things around us to be dangerous more often than not.

When someone has faults in their neuroception, they will feel isolated. Partly because they do not know who to safely approach as a friend due to misreading other people, and partly because they are not approached as often by other people due to sending out signals that conflict or do not look quite socially acceptable. The phrase *sending out the wrong signals* is really quite literal here.

Telling someone just to "act friendly," while technically accurate, is not quite enough for everyone. The person cannot show others that they are a friendly person if they do not understand the facial gestures and societal signals that indicate openness and a willingness to being approached as a safe person. For someone with a damaged or misaligned neuroception system, this must be taught.

This can be done through one-on-one therapy, personal research and study, or mingling regularly with a loved and trusted group of people who understand that this person needs help.

A man named Ravi Dykema put together a wonderful list of helpful things to keep in mind that fit nicely in the polyvagal theory regarding neuroception.

Do:

- Make eye contact when you feel safe.
- Do express with your face.
- Do modulate your voice (use expression).
- Do adjust your circumstances to feel safer – for example, move to a quieter place.
- Do adjust your focus to things that will make you feel safe, such as focusing on something familiar or comforting.
- Do play a musical instrument.
- Do try moving into social relationships instead of away, as a way to reduce slight anxiety.

Don't:

- Don't try to extend yourself physically while having a deep conversation. You're very likely to read all the cues from the other person in the wrong way.
- Don't allow yourself to become isolated. Don't seek isolation in order to feel safer. Stay connected with other people.
- Don't force yourself to interact when you aren't feeling safe enough. Bring yourself to a state of safety and then seek that interaction with other people.
- Don't discount what your gut is telling you. Pay attention, learn from what your body is telling you.
- Don't resort to fight or flight when it involves loved ones. Get to a safe place, but don't damage the relationship with your loved ones in order to do so.
- Don't allow yourself to take on a flat affect when you want the people around you to feel safe with you.
- Do not let social media or internet platforms to become a substitute for interaction with people face-to-face, or even on the phone.

- Don't assume that the worst example of someone else's behavior is their "true" self. The moments when they show peace, calm, and caretaking behavior are also just as "true" for them.

This list can be used to relearn social behaviors, to reconnect with others around you.

As the main component of the parasympathetic system, the vagus nerve is an integral part of the body's autonomic response to fear, and thus its health is paramount in being able to self soothe after a traumatic or startling event. Once the danger has passed, the vagus nerve needs to be able to tell the body this, so that it can calm itself and enter back into a state of rest.

By stimulating the vagus nerve (or waking it back up once our sympathetic nervous system has shut it down) we then flood the body with calming enzymes, sending the signal to the body that the danger is gone, and relaxation can happen again. This has been proven to alleviate stress and calm anxiety. Emotional trauma can damage, or retrain, the receptors that tell our bodies danger has passed. These traumas can trick the receptors into feeling as if the danger is still there, or that something benign is a signal of something dangerous.

When discussing the attempt to heal, or retrain, the vagus nerve, it is important to remember that the *feeling* of safety is more important than *actual* safety when it comes to signals being sent to the vagus nerve.

For example, a young boy is walking down the street outside his house minding his own business. Suddenly two large dogs appear from an alley nearby and begin to chase him. They catch him and cause him severe injury. He is only saved by the heroic actions of a passerby who steps in and fights the dogs off. Follow that same boy several months later, and he is recovered from his physical injuries. Again, he is walking down the street outside his house minding his own business when suddenly a dog approaches from an alley. This dog has its ears up, its tail in a neutral position, and sits when he sees the boy approach. The boy does not think, he just reacts, running as fast as he can in the opposite direction. The earlier traumatic event with the other pair of dogs can easily send the boy running from this second situation as well. His body has learned to interpret any dog he sees as the same life-threatening event as he experienced that first time. It is an involuntary, sympathetic reaction governed by his sympathetic nervous system. In other words, he literally cannot help himself.

The only course left is to retrain the nerves to interpret his world based on the ventral state of the vagus nerve rather than the dorsal state.

These instances so far have been based on things that happen to us, events that perhaps were no one else's fault, and certainly not of our own making.

Next, we are going to talk about something that is also not the fault of the victim, but holds a dearer, more traumatic price because it comes at the hands of someone who ought to be more caring, who ought to be loving.

## Emotional Abuse and Trauma

Sometimes faulty neuroception or an emotional trauma that changes our perceptions comes from an event that happened to us, but other times, unfortunately, emotional trauma comes directly from someone who claims to love us. When someone who ought to be taking care of us engages in emotionally abusive behavior, we can internalize it, becoming so used to their behavior that we mistakenly think it is normal and begin to judge all other behavior by that abusive measurement.

This is not your fault. This is the body's natural method of finding a way to survive. However, you can break out of the cycle of emotionally abusive behavior by first recognizing the truth, and then second, getting help to get out. These sound so easy to accomplish, and yet in reality they are not. The person who can overcome what their own body is telling them is showing courage and resilience. But first you must come to a place where you recognize that your body is just doing what it can to survive, and once that recognition takes place, you can then take charge and reteach your body what a healthy emotional state actually looks like.

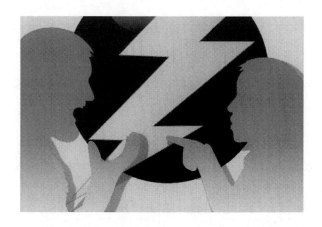

Signs of emotional abuse can be subtle, and the abuser often is a master at manipulation, using your own needs against you to create a sense of dependence on themselves.

You can spot them though, so here are some of them.

1. Humiliating behavior, negativity, and criticism in the extreme. This is not just making a mistake or wording something awkwardly, but saying things designed to humiliate or to paint you in a negative light. Nicknames that actually are cruel or demeaning – "cutie-patootie" is a cute nickname, "fatty" is not. Publicly embarrassing you, joking about things that make you look foolish or are at your expense, sarcastic remarks and then telling you that

you are being too sensitive or "just can't take a joke" when you object. Belittling you or putting down the things you are interested in, being dismissive of you or your likes or dislikes.

2. Controlling, shaming behaviors. This is often accomplished through threats and monitoring your whereabouts, both digitally and physically. Coming to your work to check up on you. I've heard of people thinking this was caring behavior, when in fact it is a sign of controlling behavior when done obsessively and to check up on whether or not you really are where you said you are going to be. This is not a sign of care, this is a sign of abuse. Lecturing and outbursts, treating you like a child and giving you direct orders rather than treating you as an equal. While acting as if you don't know to do anything on your own, they may also act as if there are certain things they have no idea how to do, so they desperately need you to do it for them.

3. Accusations, blaming others, or outright denial of things you know to be true. Jealousy, blaming you for their outbursts, lapses in judgment, or any outside problems they

may be having. Destroying things and then denying that it happened, despite proof to the contrary. Denying their abuse and possibly claiming that you are the abuser instead. Trivializing your concerns and claiming you have no sense of humor because you have been upset over things they have said in the past.

4. As the abuse continues, it will lead to emotional neglect and isolation. They will demand respect but not reciprocate. They may shut down communication, prevent you from socializing with others, or dehumanize you when you are the one doing the talking. They may come between you and family members, perhaps even offering what sounds like legitimate reasons for keeping you away from your family. At the same time, they may withhold affection from you, tune you out, or show other signs of indifference to you such as interrupting or disagreeing with you when you say you feel a certain way.

5. At the end of all this is a state of codependence. When in this state, you may feel as if you deserve this treatment, which is not true, but is hard to accept. You may feel guilty for defending yourself, and even find yourself defending

them to other people when they question this behavior. You may even be staying because they claim they cannot live without you.

You may wonder why we are talking so extensively about this sort of abuse in regard to helping yourself access the polyvagal theory of the vagus nerve. The reason is that emotional abuse changes the story you tell yourself and paints your neurological world in a way that you were not designed to see it. Again, this is not your fault. It is a biological function and up until this point, it has helped you survive. However, now you are at the point where you can see the truth, and you can get help. You may need extensive help to see the world in a healthy state again, and that is where the vagus nerve comes in. Begin that pathway to a healthy vagal state even while you are searching for help to get out of an abusive situation. This will help you start to see the world as it is meant to be, and help you gain clarity regarding the path you should follow.

# CHAPTER 3: DE-ACTIVATING

## Breaking Free

First, this chapter is not a substitute for quality therapeutic counseling from a licensed therapist. All of this ought to be seen as an aid to come alongside the help you are getting from your counselor. In fact, as we have talked about already, the polyvagal theory fully acknowledges and supports the notion that we are designed to need human intervention when we are in trauma and/or shutdown mode. You need other people.

That being said, we are living in an unhealthy state when the fight or flight response is running the show rather than the social and safety state of being. Those who have lived for a long time in a constant state of danger are left open to many other health issues as well.

When the sympathetic nervous system is activated, it floods the body with stress hormones: adrenaline, noradrenaline, cortisol, and others. While these serve us well in responding to an actual threat, the long-term effects of these hormones on the body are extensive. Conditions from mental health problems, heart disease, stroke, and high blood pressure, to gastrointestinal issues, Crohn's disease, irritable bowel, or skin problems like acne can all be attributed to long-term, chronic stress.

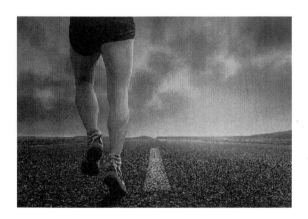

When in a heightened state, the parasympathetic system needs to produce a physical response. In order to bring the psychological state back to balance, there needs to be a physiological action. The neurons need activity – that's why deep breathing – the physical act of filling the lungs slowly and releasing the air slowly – will help. The physical act of taking a jog around the block when in fight mode… it allows the body to have a safe physiological reaction to what's going on.

Also, social connection is affected by long-term stress. A person who has been damaged to the point of being in a constant state of disassociation will have difficulty using their facial muscles to express their feelings. They can then fail to send clues of safety to others around them, and thus actually train others to respond to them as a threat. They become isolated even more then, not realizing why, creating a vicious cycle in their life.

This disassociation is the body's response to an impossible situation – when we feel trapped and powerless, we can respond by slipping into a dissociative state.

When living in a constant state of traumatic fight or flight response, we no longer accurately read other people around us.

In the next section, we will be talking about how to find your place of safety, and how to bring others into that place of safety with you.

These responses can become so embedded as children that we respond the same way even as adults, sometimes without even recognizing the true reason for those reactions.

For example, I heard a story from a mother who had a reaction to her child that puzzled her, even at the time. She had a teenager who was upset that he had overslept and missed a group outing with his friends. He came to his mother to complain. While the boy was nothing more than annoyed with himself, the mother immediately felt anger. She became upset with herself for having an angry reaction at all. Why would she have this reaction? The answer was simple – she was reacting sympathetically, literally her sympathetic nervous system throwing her into a fight response upon hearing of her son's situation even though her child was not nearly as upset as she was over it.

As she thought about the event more, she realized she had spent much of her teen years believing she had been purposely left out of things with her friend group. She spent many years feeling isolated, either ignored by family members or suffering through a lack of companions her same age. This created an automatic fight response in her when her child came to her with a scenario where he was left out, even though it was his own fault and not anything intention from his friends.

Her sympathetic nervous system was activated into fight mode, despite the fact that it was not at all appropriate to the current situation she was facing.

The process of de-activating your sympathetic neural responses will take deliberate processes but be kind to yourself. This is not about fixing you or changing something you have done wrong. This is about becoming a healthier you.

# CHAPTER 4: WINDOW OF TOLERANCE

## Your Optimal State

The vagal ladder is one way of describing where we are on the scale of safety. Another one that may resonate more with some of us is the window of tolerance.

Imagine a wave. The crest of the wave, the very top, is hyperarousal – that state where a person feels anxious, panicky, has a high startle reflex and an uneasy antsy feeling in their stomach. We have all seen it, the teenagers watching a scary movie in the dark and someone walks in on them unexpectedly. They all jump and scream, maybe knock over a lamp in the process. This is because they have been placed in a state of hypervigilance by the movie they were watching. Staying in this state for too long can also lead to chronic pain, sleeplessness, and hostility.

The bottom of the wave, the low trough, is hypo-arousal – that state where a person feels depressed, isolated, has a flat or blank affect, may feel tired all the time, and suffer from chronic fatigue. I am sure you have seen people in this state as well – perhaps after the loss of a loved one or has a major life disappointment.

In between these two extremes is a quiet middle ground, that area where we all want to live. When going through something difficult it is normal for our body to activate its defensive systems. What we don't want is to live in those defensive states for too long. We want to come back to that window of tolerance in a relatively short time where we can function in a healthy way. We can know that we are still functioning in this optimal space when we are able to engage socially, willing to reach out to those around us and ask for help.

Trauma kicks us out of this optimal state and into either the over-vigilant state, or when that is left unaddressed, may lead to us falling lower into depression. This can be demonstrated in terms of a wave-like effect. We live life in that window of tolerance but then a trauma happens, kicking us into the hyper-arousal, or activated, state. The parasympathetic system, largely the vagus nerve, does its job and brings us down from that overly activated state, but if we do not address the initial trauma, then the vagus nerve can do too good of a job, our body becoming lethargic and falling into depression, what many people describe as feeling dead inside. Left unchecked, we may unconsciously try to counter this deadness inside with risky behaviors in order to try to kick us back up to a more activated state, leading to potentially dangerous situations.

A safer way of regulating ourselves is necessary, which is why we need to learn about regulation of the vagus nerve.

## Vagal Brake

*Vagal brake* is a term that refers to the moment when a person is able to stop the sympathetic nervous system from overriding their rational thought patterns. When the vagal brake is strong, the person is able to successfully handle stress and irritation without either going into hyper-vigilance or swinging down into a depressed state. When this vagal brake is weakened or non-existent, the person is unable to process stressors, or at least is greatly hindered in handling them. This might be someone who flies off the handle at the least provocation, or they run from even minor confrontation. In severe cases, you may even see someone completely ignore a person who is trying to have a dialogue with them if there is even a hint of confrontation there.

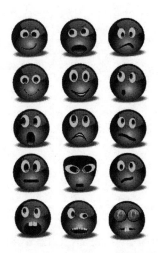

We have all been on the brink… that moment when we see the conflict in our own heart. Maybe the first simmers of an angry retort or the grinding irritation of being cut off in traffic. We have had that moment when someone jumps out at us from around a corner trying to scare us, and the first instinct is to pull an arm back and punch the person. Our fight mode has been activated through the sympathetic nervous system.

When we bite our tongue and do not respond to the angry yell, when we hold ourselves back from making a rude gesture at the driver that cut us off in traffic, when we hold back the punch from actually connecting with the nose of our friend who just startled us – those are indications of our vagal brake.

This is an important part of our neurological development, and it can save our life if we let it. I once heard the story of a young woman driving down a busy freeway in afternoon traffic – crowded, but still moving at a good clip. Her two children were buckled into their car seats in the back, a six-year-old girl and a four-year-old girl. The mom was driving along, anticipating getting home and getting the girls a snack before her husband was due back home, when all of a sudden, a blood-curdling scream erupted from the backseat. Her youngest daughter had just hit the panic button in a big way, abject terror evident in her voice. This scream is the sort that will cause every adult, parent or not parent, to jump into immediate action. It signals imminent danger, complete need for rescue, no questions asked. Immediately the mom was thrown hard into a sympathetic response.

The problem was the woman was driving her car down a crowded freeway at sixty miles per hour. Stopping was out of the question, swerving to the side of the road was definitely out of the question. Though her initial response was to grip the wheel and immediately swerve to the side of the road, the young mother was able to stop the progress of her hands just in time to keep the wheel steady. Her heart was racing, her hands were sweaty, her breath was coming in gasps. Still, she managed not to push the gas pedal down harder or slam her foot onto the brake. After the initial pulse of strong energy, she was able to signal left, pull to the next lane, and off onto the shoulder of the road to safety.

Still breathing hard, hands still sweaty, the young mother was able to turn and calmly ask her daughter what had just happened and, thankfully, was also able to appropriately respond when her daughter pointed to a harmless spider walking across her foot.

## Anxiety

Fear is a necessary neurological response. Without it, we do not recognize danger and take the appropriate reaction to either ward off that danger or escape.

Anxiety is about more than just fear though. The problem comes when our body does not recognize when that danger has passed or is not what the body assumes it to be. Our body can become trapped in that fear response, creating a sense of constant anxiety, even paranoia. Certain things can spark anxiety, growing from their gut as their dorsal vagus nerve tells their brain that something is wrong, even though the person can see that nothing around them is dangerous. This creates a sense of confusion and only adds to the anxiety.

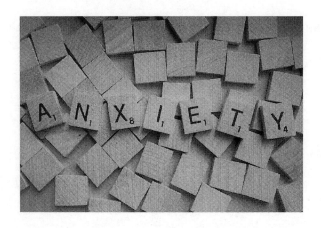

Oftentimes the person is suffering from a weakened vagal brake, having a brain that has become used to the anxiety reaction. Those nerves learn to react that way, and eventually become wired together, creating a constant sense of anxiety. Sometimes the anxiety comes from a traumatic event, and anything that reminds them of that event then triggers the anxiety.

This is when panic attacks happen. Your body is so used to the anxiety taking over that you dread its approach. Your mind is so caught up in that anxiety and fear of the anxiety itself, that now your body reacts in a panic response – your body is afraid of its own reaction and is trying to flee. This is why grounding techniques are particularly helpful with anxiety and panic attacks.

We see now what happens when someone becomes stuck in the "on" position, outside of the window of tolerance at the top of the wave we described above, in the hyperarousal state.

Anxiety is a practiced response, and so the only way to overcome it is to reteach the neural pathways to respond in a quieter fashion to triggering stimuli.

There are various methods you can do to help yourself break out of the anxiety cycle in the moment. For instance, counting backward from ten to one. It really does help. I have seen it work countless times.

Another method of breaking yourself out of the anxiety in that moment is to ground yourself in your five senses. Focus again on where your feet are touching the ground. Pick out a leaf on a nearby tree or search the ground for one of those pennies that people always drop. Try to figure out exactly what you can smell nearby. Perhaps you can smell a nearby bakery. What are they cooking that day? Perhaps you can smell a wet dog or a bed of roses in the garden. Determine what you are hearing nearby. Do you hear the sound of children playing or traffic going by? Soon you will feel the anxiety slipping away. Let it go. You will be safe without it.

Another method is to try a simple breathing exercise like this one. Breathe in for a count of four, hold your breath to the count of four, then breathe out to a count of four. After this, wait to a count of four, then repeat until you feel yourself calming again.

Sometimes the anxiety is crippling, creating a barrier for a person to lead the life they would like to lead. One thing that has been very effective for many people in this situation is to name your anxiety. Give it an actual person's name. Perhaps a character from a movie who you found particularly annoying. Welcome the now-named anxiety as if it were a real person. Invite it to walk alongside you, but not to dictate what direction you will go. Then decide where you will go next. Physically walk to that location. Practice taking charge of your anxiety as if it were a real person and you had to put them in their proper place – a place not in charge of your life.

All of these methods call for the person to live again in a state of safety. Anxiety believes itself to unsafe. You can convince it otherwise.

It is important to help ourselves have a healthy vagal brake, but in all honesty, we need each other to effectively co-regulate. We balance each other, as we will find out next.

# CHAPTER 5: CO-REGULATING

## Creating Community

Our entire society is focused on doing everything on our own. We try self-help books because we want to be able to help ourselves without relying on other people. We talk about pulling ourselves up by the bootstraps, standing on our own two feet, supporting ourselves, finding ourselves, loving ourselves, learning about ourselves, being our own safe place, self-care, self-reliance, self-awareness. What we have forgotten in all this is that we were designed to need each other.

We need co-regulation. We need to be able to find balance when we are starting to escalate, to find support when we are starting to fall into isolation, and to feel welcomed and celebrated as part of a group, part of a social circle.

We want to feel like we belong. We want to know that others around us are reacting the same way we do. This is why when something odd or upsetting happens in front of us, we look to others to see if they are having the same reaction. We want validation that what we see, or hear, or feel is the same as the others around us. Think about it – in any group of people, there is going to be a majority viewpoint and a minority viewpoint on any subject matter. In almost everything, human beings are rarely split straight down the middle in any small locale. All of us want to be surrounded by a community that thinks like we do. Thinking different says *isolation* to us, and we do not function well in social isolation. Does this mean we never reach outside our circle and try to understand someone else's viewpoint? No, because they need to feel understood as well. However, we were not designed to function in isolation. We were designed to be co-regulated.

What we then call the *vagal brake* more often than not needs other people to help co-regulate it. We can be the safety system for another person, so this section is going to focus on how we can help someone else achieve a safe state and stay there.

The following is an example of the impact of a lack of co-regulating socialization in children that leads to problems in adulthood as well as the effects of faulty neuroception.

I was recently in a meeting listening as three women were talking about their childhood struggles. Jill, Jane, and Mary (not their real names) all grew up in poverty, though Jill and Jane both had a significantly poorer upbringing than Mary did. Jill lived in a tiny house with a tarp roof and rigged electrical outlets, while Jane lived with her parents and seven siblings in a poorer country where their only dinner was routinely a handful of rice. Mary was also raised in a poor home, but at least she had food most of the time and a relatively decent house, though moving from town to town was frequent and financial struggles, sometimes grave struggles, were always present.

The three began talking, and Mary shared how she constantly has a fear of being without money. She struggles with panic when there is a bill due and she does not have enough money in the bank, and becomes agitated and anxious whenever she is faced with a new financial challenge. Neither of the other two women expressed this for themselves. Both Jill and Jane said that money does not worry them, they have a much healthier outlook on financial stressors than Mary does.

Then it came to light that both Jill and Jane had childhoods filled with strong family ties that kept them secure all through their formative years. Mary's home life was very different. Raised by parents who struggled to make emotional connections of any type with their children, Mary felt adrift during her childhood and the lack of money just made life that much more difficult. She had blamed her agitation and anxiety on the lack of money, when in fact her fears more likely came from a lack of social bonding with those who were responsible for her emotional security.

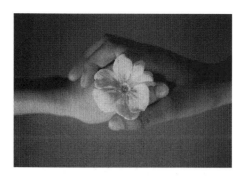

In this case, the polyvagal theory comes into play in that Mary needed that social bonding, that connection with someone to help her regulate her state of being. The other two women had that social bonding which gave them security even through very difficult times. This is called co-regulating, and it is a vital part of maintaining a healthy vagal state. By not having this as a child, Mary was left in some part functioning in a fight-or-flight state and thus was close to panic at the slightest threat to her financial status – her sense of security.

When helping someone out of that lowered vagal state, the calming voice, the non-confrontational eyes with the corners crinkled in a friendly smile, the body posture not towering over them and not demanding anything from them are essential.

These are cues to safety that the other person can use to pull himself up from that slide into an even lower state.

People without a safety system will have a feeling of danger when they are still. Being still (not frozen, but purposeful stillness) is a function of being safe. You are free to be still with someone only when you feel safe with them. For people who are "down the ladder," being bored or still is intolerable. With this in mind, we can give them something to do. It seems simple, but offering to go for a walk, giving the restless, activated student an active errand to run, or requiring an action from the small child ready to throw a tantrum. These can and do help to enable the vagal brake.

✱ ✱ ✱

Our goal in interacting with those around us should be to create a state of safety. When someone is struggling with this, we need to help them come back to a safe state. We can do this by meeting them where they are. Name what they are experiencing. Do not contradict or act as if you are in a different state, and do not meet them with a sense of scorn. They are reacting to something they see as a threat, so validate that feeling rather than try to contradict it. Then bring them back to a place of social engagement by talking quietly or better yet, by listening completely.

Sometimes all you can do is be there for them and wait until they no longer feel threatened.

Trying to reason with someone who is frozen is not going to work. They are shut down and logic does not get through. They may only understand quiet presence.

So often when helping another person, we want to be proactive. We hear a loved one's complaint or notice their aggravation and their emotional wounds, and we instinctively are kicked into that sympathetic mode ourselves. We want to confront the person that hurt them, or get up and move, perhaps we want to immediately begin offering a solution to their trauma. These are all autonomic responses of our own. Remember that when your sympathetic system is engaged, because it is a neurological process, we feel an instinctual need to physically move, to fight the threat, to run from the danger. But in this case, that is not what will help the other person the most. The best therapy for another person's emotional upheaval is just to be in the presence of a trusted loved one. You can do more for that person by just sitting quietly and listening to them than by remaining activated and attempting to drive home some solution.

This concept also has implications for those working in the therapy field, or even ministers and pastors, or parents. We have seen how living in a sympathetically activated state can be detrimental to our health, both physically and emotionally. Therapists, ministers, pastors, nurses … really anyone in a field that requires them to be social therapists of some sort, they are all prone to extreme burn out. Perhaps this is why - they remain activated sympathetically all the time. There will be times when they absolutely need to be in their sympathetic state, but if they can switch back to just being the trusted individual in that person's life, just being there without the need to try to push through to a solution for that person, then they have actually accomplished much of the solution they were hoping to find.

Further, those around us need us to be a safe person for them, but too often people misunderstand *what being a safe person* means. It does not mean feeling their pain. It does not mean feeling sorry for them.

Being a safe person does mean hearing their pain without being hurt by it. It means having compassion *without* feeling their pain. It means being strong enough to not be hurt by what that person is telling you or what they have experienced. Perhaps this is why a child will tell a teacher or trusted counselor something that happened to them rather than a parent. It explains why we instinctively hold back from sharing things with our closest family members and sometimes will share those things with strangers instead.

We can be the strong but compassionate burden bearers in our loved ones' lives. With that in mind, the following sections deal with what a safe environment might look like in the various social communities we may find ourselves in.

If we make a practice of fostering feelings of safety in everyone around us, we have the key to help them develop into more healthy individuals, thus creating a safer environment for everyone.

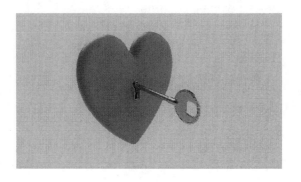

## Safety At Home

I have heard it said that humans were designed to go through life nestled in a warm and cozy nest of emotional bondedness and social connectedness. Imagine if that were true of our homes. People should find safety at home. Acceptance, reassurance, openness without judgment, listening in order to understand rather than listening to answer. Home in particular needs to be a place where everyone feels safe to disagree if necessary. Storming out, or becoming obviously hurt if a child does not want to reveal their innermost thoughts to a parent does not create a sense of safety in that child. This actually creates the opposite reaction, teaching the child that the parent is not a safe person to confide in. Even becoming activated for the sake of the other person, demanding to be allowed to fix the situation, or ranting in that person's stead, can all create a sense of danger in regards to confiding in that person.

Creating safety at home means being free to share or not share, to be close or to be spending time alone without judgment over either one. Safety at home should represent the ultimate freedom and sense of belonging, in community with one another.

## Safety At School

In order for children to learn, they need to feel safe. Remember, once the sympathetic nervous system has been activated, cognition is lowered. Kids literally cannot think clearly when their system is activated to identify and neutralize threats in their environment. That child who is unable to focus may have started their day being yelled at by their parents for something the night before. Or worse, they had to get themselves up and to school on their own because their parent or guardian was not present for any number of reasons.

Perhaps they had to walk to school. Some children arrive at school after having walked through all sorts of dangerous situations. For many children, just the bus ride to school is rife with tension.

These kids need a safe place at school. They need to know that someone will listen. They need to know that the teachers and administration understand who they are and want to connect with them as people rather than as a student number or a grade in a grade book.

Often the best thing is awareness. When teachers and administrators are aware of the potential problems, they can be present for each child in a meaningful way, when that child needs them. Strategies such as carrying emotion and needs cards so a child can use them when he is unable to articulate his own needs or emotions.

## Safety At Places Of Worship

These should be sanctuaries of refuge, places to go where we can find shelter from life's troubles. The church environment can be enhanced by leadership who understands that everyone coming in through their front doors has different needs. Churches are places where a wide variety of people come together for a joint goal. Because of this variety, there are going to be many different kinds of issues presenting themselves. Having people on hand who can help with someone in a specific need is always good. I know some churches have a nurse on call during each service in case someone has a medical emergency. Perhaps they could have a therapist volunteer or someone who works in counseling be available to help someone who comes in showing distress.

Perhaps the better thing would be to have some training open to all members on how to better approach the vulnerable people in their community who come to them for help.

## Safety At Work

Work can be a place filled with danger for many people. Looming deadlines, the expectations of bosses, co-workers depending on us or not doing their own fair share of the workload. All of these cause stress and create a difficult work environment.

Deadlines can be intimidating. Pressure to get more done and to get it done more effectively build up with time. Providing a safe workplace does not have to come at the sacrifice of productiveness. People create more when in a place of safety. Their cognition is higher, their capacity for work is greater when they are under less stress.   We can create safety everywhere we go.

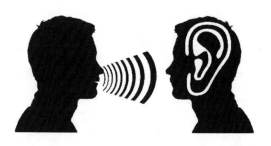

**Practice Listening**

We can help those around us by practicing listening, and with that in mind, I've gathered a list of ways we can consider when determining whether or not we are a good listener ourselves.

1. Listen to understand, not to respond. It seems counterintuitive at first but listening to someone else in sincerity means not being distracted by what you want to say to them next. It means setting aside your own opinions for the moment and listening in order to hear their heart.
2. While you should listen to understand, you also want to ask questions to clarify. Show that you are engaged in what they are saying by asking them if you are understanding correctly. Perhaps ask if they mean one of two options or ask them if that is what they are trying to say. Be clear that you are not asking in order to judge, but that you are asking in order to understand fully.
3. In the pursuit of clarity, asking questions to understand, remember that you cannot drag someone else up the polyvagal ladder. Honor their dignity by accepting that they have their own choices to make and will need to go

through the process of pulling themselves up to a higher state. You may be the listening partner, but you cannot do the work for them.

4. Listen for their needs while putting aside your own needs. I have sometimes been in the position where I am listening to someone present a problem that they are struggling with only to have the nearly uncontrollable urge to fix their issue. I feel as if I "need" to offer a solution and be heard. When this happens, I am no longer hearing them. Rather, if I insist on telling them the solution that I believe is correct, then I am trying to have my own need met. It has ceased to be about helping them and has become an exercise to help myself instead, to fulfill that need I have to be a help. This may seem like a sincere desire to help the other person, but once I put my own needs first, I cease to be a help to them. When this happens, they automatically become the co-regulator for me, and if they are already in an unstable state as well, then that co-regulating is ineffective. Do not flip on the person trying to get help. Remain outside yourself for the moment, deny yourself the need to fix

something, and just be present for the other person for a little while.
5. Try to listen even if the other person is not making sense at that moment. This may seem to contradict the point about asking for clarification, but it is really just a branch of that. Asking for clarity is different than making a judgment regarding whether or not their feelings or their solution makes sense at the time. If they ask for advice, that is the time to give the advice. Wait until they are ready for advice before giving it, and do not make any judgments regarding whether or not their currently voiced interpretation of the situation, or their solution makes any sense.
6. Trust that the other person can come to their own solution. Do not assume that if they are coming to you, then you are required to offer some sort of wisdom or a piece of advice or a call to action. Trust that they have the answer inside themselves, and if they do not, and want your advice, then they will ask for it.
7. Honor their choices and their opinions. If they are upset or are expressing an opinion you do not agree with, you

do not have to listen in order to convince them they are wrong. They are only asking you to listen. Listen to understand comes in to play here again. You may find out that there is a motivation behind their opinion or choice that you did not fully comprehend at first. Sometimes that motivation brings to light some facts you were not aware of, and perhaps you would find yourself in agreement instead of being on opposite sides. Regardless, the listener is not present to change the other person. The listener is only present. Be that present person for your friend or loved one.

Becoming a good listener does take practice. Even the most compassionate person wants to help, and it takes practice to sit quietly and feel as if you are doing nothing to help. However, the exercise of listening quietly is in itself a help. Often that is all the other person needs. You will start to see them change, to climb up that vagal ladder, to enter again into their optimal window of tolerance. Let them talk themselves down. You are there to figuratively hold their hand during that process. You are not there to take the steps for them.

Someone once told me that many years ago she was going through the most traumatic experience of her life. She did not know how she was going to hold herself together. Yet, to this day, many years later, there is one person who stood out as having helped her through this great trauma in her life. Many people were supportive, but this one person stood out in the story because of what she did *not* do. She did not speak. She was only present for this woman. She offered no words of wisdom. She offered no solution. She offered no soft words of comfort. She only listened, sitting quietly, or offering a hug when she sensed the need. Yet the woman telling me this story said that other lady helped her in a profound way, such that it stands out to her still to this day. So profound, and yet nothing was said. Apparently being a passive listener is anything but passive.

# CHAPTER 6: STORIES WE TELL OURSELVES

## Your Story and Your State

People are storytellers. We view the world around us as a narrative, telling ourselves stories that fit the stimuli we take in moment by moment. Those stories may be mostly true, or mostly false. They may be part of an attempt to lie to ourselves, or part of our way of preserving our own mental sanity. These stories shape our perception of the situations we find ourselves in, the people we interact with on a daily basis, and the path forward that we see in life. No matter what, they are an integral part of our daily thought life, and those stories we tell ourselves are based on the information gathered through the vagus nerve.

Have you ever wondered why two people can walk into a room full of strangers, and while one sees friendly faces of potential friends, the other sees faces of judgment and criticism, the faces of potential enemies?

I heard one woman say that sometimes she would walk into a room and feel judged by everyone there. She just knew that every person looking at her was being critical of her clothes, her weight, her makeup, everything about her. She went on to say that whenever she did that, she would stop, turn around and go back out, and ask herself why she was feeling so self-conscious.

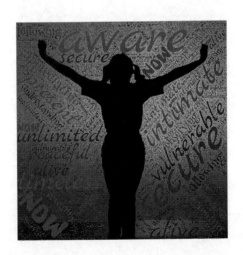

She would then talk herself down from that perception, reminding herself that people are not always thinking of her, and they most likely have their own troubles on their mind. Most likely people are not thinking of her at all, and certainly not in such a negative light. There was no reason for her to be so insecure or self-conscious. She would then turn back and enter the room, finding that her feelings of judgment coming from the others in the room had all dissipated.

The above is an example of the state of your body determining your brain's story. Your body takes in information from its surroundings, and then creates a story based on that information, including its perception of other people. That story changes based on which state of being you are existing in at the time.

First, we will define the three states again. We have named them so far in this narrative, but let's put them in order now again. The highest, healthiest state is the safe/social state, or ventral – that state where we feel safe and we are able to be social. The second state is sympathetic response to danger – that state where we are reacting instinctively to something our body is telling us is a threat, a danger, either by fighting it or fleeing from it. The third and final is the dorsal state – in which we no longer are thinking at all, unable to connect, isolated, shut down.

In the ventral state, we are able to think clearly about others, versus when we are in the sympathetic state where we are much more likely to misinterpret the signals we are getting from those around us. People are more likely to be seen as an enemy rather than a friend trying to help. Biologically our body is just trying to keep us alive when in the sympathetic state, but n the dorsal state, others have essentially ceased to exist. We feel alone because we have disconnected from the world around us.

As an example, let's look at a specific hypothetical case. Imagine a child who is raised by an emotionally absent father and a mother who had retreated into an emotional shut-down state herself as a means of securing her own emotional preservation.

As a child, he will feel isolated, suffering through what he sees as rejection, and eventually interpreting everything as a negative, even though it may not be intended that way.

As an adult, he has disconnected himself, no longer realizing the proper affect for promoting healthy relationships. Having a vagus nerve that has not had much input from facial muscles means it considers anything in the face as a danger sign. Anything out of the ordinary can be interpreted as dangerous then.

While facial expressions can be learned based on watching other people, to people who naturally emote in their face, his expressions may look fake. Now he unknowingly signals to others that he is a fake person, seeming to be hiding something. He begins to look like a threat to others around him, when in fact he feels the emotions the same as others and wants to be friends. Here we see another example of safety being about perception, not about reality, even in the case of people who normally correctly read social cues. The people around him were perceiving danger signals (albeit unconsciously) although no danger existed in this case.

His environment tells him one thing, the reactions he sees from others around him tells him another thing. His brain takes all those bits of information and forms a story from them. At this point in his life, he is telling a story to himself that involves people not liking him very much, not trusting him. He starts to see himself as flawed, unworthy. He does not really know why, just that every interaction seems to be negative, if there are any interactions at all. Negative thoughts abound. His brain tells him that people are talking about him behind his back, they are casting judgment on him, they are not accepting him or they are laughing at him. His heart is heavy, depression is settling in.

Then one day he finds out that the vagus nerve seems to learn from its environment. It takes in information from the facial expressions of his own body, sending signals of safety to his own heart and mind. What could he lose? He may as well try it and see.

Next time he is in a crowd, he practices real expressions of what he truly feels – rather than the wide-eyed expressions he thought signaled interest in what the other person was saying, he tried crinkling the corners of his eyes, living in happy thoughts, allowing feelings of warmth toward people he genuinely knows and enjoys. He concentrates on staying present in his mind, not letting his thoughts wander off while talking to someone.

Suddenly, in the midst of the social experiment, he realizes that his mind is not telling him negative stories anymore. His mind is instead content, quiet. There are no thoughts of someone being angry with him or another person perhaps being offended.

Looking back, he can see that in reality the same amount of people talked to him as the last time. He had roughly the same amount of social engagement. The difference was that he felt a part of it more this time. He felt like he belonged. His brain did not interpret anyone as talking bad about him. He did not suspect anyone of judging him or laughing at him. He could clearly differentiate between normal body language versus the language of rejection. The only thing that had changed was the story his own brain was telling himself, based solely on changing his own expressions.

It is important to recognize that some of that storytelling part of our brain is neurological. At times we try to change the story in our brain without recognizing the neurological component. We are designed as neurological beings, and that part of our brain is affected literally by our neurons – over a hundred thousand of those neurons exist. Imagine the impact of such a great number of neurons on the brain, telling it stories, interpreting the world for us, helping to shape the perception of everything we see and everyone we know.

Changing the interpretation of the input your brain is getting from that vagus nerve is crucial to re-telling our own story, and telling ourselves a balanced story as we walk through each day is crucial to remaining in a connected, safe, and social state with ourselves, and with those around us.

Next, we will explore a few ways to help ourselves learn to retell that story.

# CHAPTER 7: SOMATIC EXPERIENCING

## Somatic Experiencing And The Polyvagal Theory

So often we think of our mind and our brain as being two separate entities. We do not think of them as connected, but they are. When we experience the term *psychology,* we think of it as wholly separate from anything biological in our bodies.

This is a mistake. Our bodies are woven together with our emotional senses. One therapeutic method that is affected by the polyvagal theory is somatic mindfulness.

**Somatic mindfulness** - *This kind of therapeutic work softens and reduces the hypervigilant threat response and hyperarousal in the nervous system.*

Somatic mindfulness is all about integrating the mind and the body, finally fully understanding the capacity of the mind to impact the body, and the body to impact the mind. It is about that moment you realize that your mind is reacting to something that your body is sensing and that you can act immediately to reassure your body, thus reassuring your mind as well.

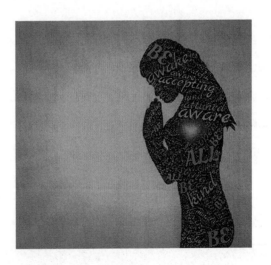

One way to get to somatic mindfulness is to go through somatic experiencing. This is a specific type of therapy that trains the patient to track the sensations coming through their body, and how to interpret those experiences correctly in relation to what they tell the mind. This may include breathing techniques, voice work, exercise, dance, or other things.

Somatic mindfulness is simply getting to the place where you know what your body is telling you. Being aware of what your senses are experiencing on a deep level. Being mindful of your body means you pay attention when your gut is telling you something, it means recognizing the signs of an impending panic attack, sensing when your anger is mounting to a dangerous level, being able to see that something is creating havoc in your body and being aware enough to want to take action before that something boils over.

Somatic mindfulness is exemplified in the woman we mentioned in the previous chapter who recognized her own self-consciousness as being a reaction to signals her body was sending and was not necessarily indicative of the reality of the people in the room. She did not voice this as being part of somatic experience, but she understood it on a deep level.

Somatic experiencing is all about taking that next step. Once you have recognized that something is happening to trigger your sympathetic, subconscious reaction center, then the next step is making a conscious effort to take a physical action instead. Again, recalling the woman in the previous chapter, she took a physical action – walking back out of the room – and used that moment to talk herself back into a healthier mental state.

Before your subconscious takes that action then, you need to counter it with a conscious effort. Instead of yelling at that other person in anger, count to ten. Instead of running out of the room in fear of a large crowd, ground yourself by focusing on where your feet touch the floor, for instance.

Somatic experiencing is part of telling your brain a new story, letting the sensations around you be interpreted in a healthier way, and coming to a point where your body and mind can tell a more accurate story to each other.

# CHAPTER 8: PLAY IN A POLYVAGAL WORLD

## Playing In A Polyvagal World

Did you know that play has a definition? According to play expert, Dr. Peter Gray, in order to qualify as truly play, it must have these five characteristics:

- An activity that is chosen on your own and directed on your own
- Engaged in for the sake of the activity and not for some reward
- Includes some sort of structure or set of rules
- Employs an imaginary element of some kind
- Be done in an alert, conscious frame of mind

Based on those criteria, much of what we do these days is not truly considered play.

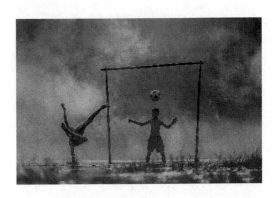

For many years, children were allowed to play on their own, but now we have changed all that. Children spend most of their time either in school, doing homework, or in some sort of extracurricular activity that the parents have deemed important. I remember as a child I used to walk outside and encounter other children playing all the time, but now children go outside to be met with silent streets. No one has time to go outside and play in their yards because they are too busy being shuttled to ballet, art class, piano lessons, after-school activities, organized sports, something. Always something else. While these activities alone would not be a problem, it is the fact that they have now so completely taken over children's lives to the detriment of free time.

Parents feel the need to supervise every moment of their child's day, not only watching them constantly, but also directing them in all of those activities. There are seemingly no independent moments for children anymore, and certainly nothing that involves risk. I have seen parents upset at their child for climbing a tree, when in fact, tree climbing is a time-honored activity that ought to be enjoyed by every child. We have lost the notion of free play.

How does this relate to the polyvagal theory, you might ask? Well, by structuring our children's day to the last minute, every day, we have set up a framework for them to grow up in. Their neural development is still happening during these years, and they are now only experiencing rigid structure, rules placed on them by someone else, play directed not by themselves but by some outward force. And all activities in a completely safe environment, no risks involved anywhere.

You may ask why any of that might bear on the neurological development. As the polyvagal theory teaches, if we can train our vagus pathways to respond more appropriately to situations that have caused us anxiety in the past, then it stands to reason that we can train our neurological pathways to only feel safe in a structured environment. By not allowing our children to have adequate time to play freely, we have trained them that they are only safe in structured moments. Imagine then when the child turns into an adult and no one is telling them every step to take, every rule they must follow. Many of us do not need to imagine it now, because it is exactly what we felt when we became that adult ourselves.

I mentioned risk for a reason as well. Growing up in an environment where you are never in any sort of self-directed risky situation means you will never learn that you have the capacity to survive these minor risks. Here I am not talking about purposely living in a constant state of fear or actual danger, but rather just allowing your child to do things that involve minor risk. Climbing a tree comes to mind. Wrestling with other kids, riding a bike, swinging from a tree swing. These things prove to the child that they can handle minor fear, that they can survive a certain amount of risk and they can take charge of their own environment.

These are vital lessons to learn as children, and the lack of these lessons carries on into adulthood. A child who does not know how to problem solve in freestyle play will be an adult who does not know how to problem solve on the job.

Perhaps this lack of play as children has also contributed to the rise in anxiety in adults in recent years. Imagine entering adulthood feeling completely unprepared and having no idea how to prepare oneself. Not even knowing what you are lacking in so you can go out and teach it to yourself. We have all this technology at our fingertips, yet the only thing we really need to do is use our imaginations in free play time.

I read of one community that may have found a solution to this issue. They have a community play time during which families bring their children specifically for unstructured play time. The only structure allowed is the meeting time and the agreed-upon playground, and an adult or two to provide light supervision in case of real emergencies and to prevent truly life-threatening risky behavior. Otherwise, children from kindergarten through fifth grade are allowed to freely roam, playing whatever games they choose, and interacting with whomever they wish in that environment.

Free play is an integral part of the story we tell ourselves as adults. It has an impact on what we perceive about our own abilities, and the dangers existing in our surroundings. Free play tells us what we are truly capable of and forces us to stretch our minds and bodies to overcome obstacles and solve problems.

Let's bring free play back into our world.

# CHAPTER 9: MUSIC

## The Role of Music in the Polyvagal Theory

Music paints a picture of the world around us and uploads it directly to our brain. It can take us from scared, frozen in fear, to energized and activated. It can make us sad or happy, raise us to heights of triumph or drag us down to the depths of defeat and sorrow. It makes sense then that music can have a direct impact on our perceived state of being as affected by our vagus nerve.

A musical score with discordant notes in a minor key, an unsteady rhythm, all sends signals of danger to our brain. In the same way, a piece of music that is either very low pitched or in contrast is very high pitched can send danger signals. Perhaps this is why we use deep-toned sounds for foghorns as warning signals, but we also react to a baby's high-pitched scream as a sign that immediate parental action is required.

Music that runs too fast can make us feel uneasy, as if we are in danger of missing important information, but music that runs too slow can give the impression that the message is not coming across quickly enough.

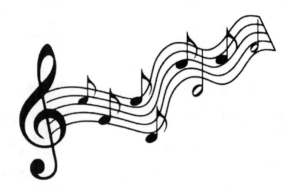

Not much study has been done surrounding music and how it may or may not impact our natural sense of safety, but in August 2015, one article was published that may shed some insight on this process.

The conductors of the experiment wanted to find out what brought on the most sense of safety: silence, sounds of nature, or music. In essence, they wanted to find out if music could trigger a sense of safety.

Their study came away with several conclusions and some surprising findings, one of which being that a cappella music was seen as slightly more dangerous than straight instrumental music. Their guess about this finding was that perhaps it was because voice music carries a bit more variability and unpredictability than the instrumental would have. Perhaps also it could be explained by the notion of human voices raised in unison brings with it a sense of urgency or a call to action, unlike non-voiced instrumental music.

One of the two main focuses of the study was to find out if music holds fewer danger signals than nature sounds and silence. The study showed that yes, music was seen as an indicator of safety. This may tell us that music provides an information system that tells the body things about its environment. Simple music without much movement was also seen as more dangerous or stress-inducing than music more complex and faster. Music that was too fast was seen as a stressor or danger signal as well.

It was interesting to note that each person's optimal speed and intensity of music was different.

Through this, we can see that music could be an important part of overcoming trauma and sustaining a healthy mind and body relationship.

Music has a direct impact on the cranial muscles of the face, meaning the music itself helps to stimulate the vagus nerve and teaches our body how to react to the world around us.

We can also use music to bring us into a healthier state of mind. With today's technology, you can find music to fit every need simply by doing a simple search in your internet browser.

Think of how music can help soothe the mind of an autistic person, offering order and structure, and perhaps a sense of safety in the midst of a world that they see as bombarding them with too much chaotic information at all times.

That same sort of soothing can be for you too.

# CHAPTER 10: SOCIAL MEDIA

## Vagus Nerve And Social Media

Social media is a part of our lives now. There is no going back, and I doubt that we ought to even try. Social media says to our brains that we are being social, but are we? Are we connecting on that neurological level?

Recent studies have found that higher use of social media actually correlates with higher feelings of isolation among teenagers. This tells me that being on social media does not always tell your body that you are in a community of other people, that you are being accepted and welcomed in and responded to.

Sometimes people intentionally inflate their followers or their friends list on whatever social media platform they prefer. They are trying to create a crowd in the hopes that the more numbers they see, the more they will feel as if they are in a community with other people. Contrary to their intentions, all this does is inflate their isolation. The numbers do not have arms to reach out, and subconsciously we realize this.

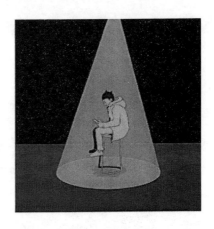

Can we have meaningful relationships online? Yes, I believe so. There are anecdotes all around us of people who have deep and satisfying relationships with people they have met online. Those friends are just as much friends as people we know offline. The difference is that in trying to create a crowd, we wind up relying on numbers rather than real conversation. This is part of the story we tell ourselves again. When a person begins to rely on the numbers they see revolving around their social media platform, then social connection becomes all about a shallow reward-based system. Make a post or share a picture that gets likes, and then interpret that as the reward, creating an entire relationship around the clicking of a button.

As much as it is true online, you can feel terribly alone standing in a crowd of people who are physically present with you. Having a crowd around you means nothing if no one is there with you, being present with you and joining in with you. Even a stranger who pauses to notice you will be enough to ease some of that loneliness when in a physical crowd.

Just as in your offline life, having a few close friends who really understand you and take time to talk and interact with you on a deeper basis is what will create that feeling of community that you long for. The problem with social media that I see is that it relies so heavily on numbers rather than any meaningful connection.

Secondarily, another problem with social media is that you can put up an image of yourself that is only a partial image, or is airbrushed, sometimes literally. What you put on those social media platforms can be only the best of yourself, only the brightest, only the perfect. And when people respond positively to that, you are unconsciously teaching yourself that people only like the best parts of you. This does not create a trusting relationship, and we instinctively know it. This creates a social connection based on an image, a fake image, and that is a very lonely thing indeed.

You can change this. You can create an online sense of community as well as an offline one. I do believe it is better to have that offline connection though as well. Don't isolate yourself from those physically with you. We all need that physical interaction, so do not deprive yourself of that. We are finding out that our very neurons cry out for that connection with other people.

# CHAPTER 11: CREATE SAFETY

## Safe and Social

After all this, your sense of well-being and safety is up to you. You can choose to reach out to get help from others. You can surround yourself with things that help you stay in that optimal state. You can create the story that you tell yourself.

Creating safety around yourself will bring you back into a more balanced perspective on life, and to a place of more healthful living.

Be creative – write. You do not have to be good at it, you just need to write. Put the feelings down on paper and let them speak for themselves now. Leave those feelings there as you are writing them down. The physical act of writing can have a deep impact on your sense of safety, allowing an outlet for the muscles to release some of that energy.

Find a focus – distract yourself from the anxiety by looking for something specific in your environment. Look for a pebble, a leaf, a flower, find the clouds, or look for something blue. Be creative. Become a hunter of that object or color.

The human voice can sometimes kickstart us into our ventral system. Listen to a podcast or an inspirational message. Listen to the soothing voice of a narrator reading a favorite book, or a new book we have never read.

Get grounded: focus on the floor under your feet, the armrests under your arms, the seat under your seat. Feel the breeze on your face, let your body feel cold or hot, feel the hair move on your head. Concentrate on what your eyes see, focus in on what your ears are hearing, identify some smells in your environment.

Remember that the nervous system's automatic responses require movement. The need to move is built into us, and so listen to your body. Accept what your body is telling you. Let your body respond to that need but redirect it to a safe activity.

When we create safety for ourselves, we will be better equipped to create safety for those around us as well.

# PART THREE

In the next section we will be looking more closely at Autism Spectrum Disorder, the various ways it affects individuals, and how the Polyvagal Theory may be helping to create safety and social connection among a group of people who have a unique struggle in this area.

# CHAPTER 1: POLYVAGAL AND AUTISM

## Autism Spectrum Disorder

Autism is a large and complex disorder that spans an entire spectrum, to the point that one definition for autism cannot really be summed up in totality in just one sentence. However, generally speaking, autism is a sensory disorder, affecting different individuals to different degrees and manifesting in different ways for each individual.

In the United States alone, one in fifty-nine children are autistic, with one in thirty-seven boys and one in one hundred-fifty-one girls, and the numbers of diagnoses seem to be going up. Whether this is due to a rising incidence of the condition or rising awareness is not yet completely known. Most of these children are not diagnosed until after the age of four, although there have been cases of children as young as two years old being diagnosed.

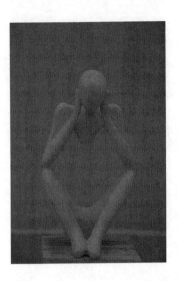

Being a spectrum disorder means there is a range of symptoms affecting social and communication skills, as well as motor and language skills to some degree – sometimes greater, sometimes less.

Often the autistic individual sees social cues as danger signs rather than invitations to engage, or they could completely lack those social instincts needed to navigate in a social world. They may see a hug as an attack, a smile as a grimace, or an exuberant greeting as a grating intrusion on their sense of peace.

In recent years though there has been some progress made on figuring out what may be the cause of or contributing factors to autism.

One thing that is said now to be a factor is inflammation and immune problems – specifically neuro-inflammation and neuro-immune abnormalities. If the vagus nerve helps to reduce inflammation, perhaps some people with autism will be receiving help in a short while, but that is the neurological, biological part of the struggle with autism. We are going to focus now on the connection between the mind and the body, and how it relates to the world of the autistic person.

## Mind-body Connection

However, one thing that is becoming more apparent is that a method of therapy called mind-body connectedness is showing promise in the autistic world.

On a daily deep level, those with autism contend with a problem connecting their mind to their body and letting it stay there. The noise that surrounds them is overwhelming, causing their senses to overload. The only relief they have is through withdrawal. Perhaps we can offer some relief in some other way.

Those on the spectrum have a problem recognizing the way their body feels in a safe state. Rather than an inability to recognize safety physically, though that is also often present, this is the inability to understand that their state of mind is safe. It does not seem safe to them, so they need added reinforcement to recognize that state and allow their bodies to stay in it. Think of it this way – if you are born within a state of fight or flight, your body will come to recognize that as what is your normal. Anything outside that normal becomes a sign of danger. Bring that body to a quiet, calm state, and those neurons will fire off warnings and danger signals, thinking there is some sort of danger to be fought off.

One thing to remember, first, is that the goal for anyone on the autism spectrum is not to become *normal*, or the same as most people around them. They are normal already, just their normal.

Their senses become overwhelmed, but this does not indicate that their senses are wrong. The person with autism has heightened sensitivity, but that also translates into heightened perception, heightened appreciation for beauty or music, a heightened ability to see or hear things that slip past other people.

Our society is not "autism friendly". Our society is not built in a way that is sensitive to those with sensory disabilities. There is always some noise or flashing lights, weird smells, bright colors, fast-moving crowds or traffic, then we place the autistic person in numerous social settings that are dependent on only instincts. They are left in a crowd wondering where the social engagement manual was hidden because they didn't get to read it. They are placed in schools where other kids seem to know exactly how to act instinctively, while they are left alone to struggle through mistake after mistake. They are placed in social settings where they can see a hierarchy exists but they have no idea how to function within that hierarchy. This would be absolutely terrifying, and it is no wonder they often shut down.

Even with all this, there is no reason to bring them to a state that looks like everyone else. What they most need is to be brought into a state where they are more comfortable, a place where they can be safe and happy in their own body, whatever that state looks like. The individual with autism will have his or her own happy optimal state, and that is what the caregiver or therapist or loved one should focus on helping them find.

Polyvagal theory approaches autism from a different direction than many other treatments and therapy models. It looks at the person's neurological state and assumes that something has caused this person's biology to immobilize them, perhaps from birth. Immobilization is a very real, very biological thing. We know that this state exists now. It is further than just freezing, or even dissociation. It is immobilization where a person literally cannot move. They cannot access their body in a functional state, and it is happening to them on a neurological level. The autistic person may have something happening to his body that he cannot control. Instead, it has been taken over by the sympathetic nervous system.

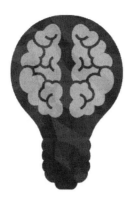

This is why therapy from a polyvagal viewpoint will approach the body of the person on the spectrum first. The belief is that the autistic person is so disconnected from their body that they cannot control it sometimes. They cannot control the slide into a meltdown, and they do not know how to keep themselves in that safe space. There is also much evidence that says they do not recognize a safe space when it does happen. Even a state of stillness can be seen as a threat to the autistic person. Perhaps they have only ever experienced stillness as a response to perceived danger, their body having always interpreted the stimuli around them as signals of danger. They need to be taught that stillness can happen in safety as well.

Researchers used to believe that the brain reaches a certain point and never changes after that, but more recent studies have called that conclusion into question. Now the science of neuroplasticity is giving us indications that the brain can change and grow, even into adulthood.

How does this impact autism? This thought impacts autism in that we now believe the autistic brain can change, be taught to tolerate sensory stimuli, at least to a better degree than they are used to. This can lead to more comfort for the person living with autism, as well as provide more weapons for their arsenal in combatting difficult, complex social issues. While we do not want to change who they are, we do wish to give them some relief from their isolation. They may feel betrayed by their body. They can learn that they do not have to feel betrayed anymore, but instead can come into unity with their body, and bring it to a place of safety.

There are some therapies that focus on this specifically. Some chiropractors have also seen improvement when working with autistic children.

The point of this sort of therapy is to get yourself into a safe and open position and learn that there is no danger there. For the sake of your loved one with autism, you are tasked with creating that safety for them when they are doing an exercise like this.

Allow them to have space, trust that they can improve, trust that they have the ability to think things through on their own. Let them have that moment to climb up the vagal ladder on their own, while you create a safe space around them for them to accomplish this goal.

When working with an autistic child, the activities to enhance the brain-body connection can be simple.

I have seen a teacher cut out dinosaur shapes for a child who loved dinosaurs to use in learning his place values for math. She made different sizes, then baby dinosaurs, and lined them up to each represent different place values. This is a form of brain-body connection because the child could manipulate the dinosaurs and connect that physical touch with a learned fact. He was connecting his body to his mind.

Mind-body therapies include things like meditation, prayer, guided imagery, biofeedback, yoga, and cognitive behavioral therapy.

In the next chapters, we are going to discuss a few of these therapies and how they fit in to the polyvagal theory for creating a safe place for the autistic individual to function within society.

# CHAPTER 2: COGNITIVE BEHAVIORAL THERAPY

This form of therapy often takes the approach of writing negative, destructive, or dysfunctional thought processes down in a journal, then devising healthier thought patterns, often with the help of a therapist. Cognitive behavioral therapy can be carried out alone though if needed or preferred.

This is also called cognitive restructuring and is part of the idea that your brain can be taught to renew itself, to change its thought patterns.

Take the case of the autistic teenaged boy named John (not his real name). John comes to his parents, upset that he has seen someone they know showing his parents a picture of his neurotypical sister as she's standing with a group of her friends. His thoughts are that no one seems to ever care enough about him, or think he's worthy of, a nice candid picture.

His parents instruct him to sit down and write out his thoughts and they will discuss them with him if he'd like once he's through. Through this process, he writes that he is afraid people don't like him because they don't show him as much attention as they show his sister. As he writes, his mind calms. He is able to picture the photo he saw and in that moment he also realizes that the person taking the picture showing his sister also had their child in the frame. Perhaps they were taking a picture of their own child, and it had nothing to do with his sister specifically. Upon coming to that realization, John was able to think more calmly about the situation and see that perhaps he was overreacting.

Through this we see the cognitive pattern coming to light, simply through the process of writing it down. Of course, this assumes that the autistic individual has the capacity to write.

This exercise dovetails well with the polyvagal theory in that it uses a physical action to help bring a person back closer to a safe and social state.

In order to practice this method yourself, here are some steps to follow.

First, help yourself reach a state of calm. Use some of the breathing techniques mentioned here in this book, or your own.

Second, identify the situation. Describe to yourself what created the issue in your mind in the first place.

Third, analyze your mood during the encounter. This is not referring to specific thoughts, but how you were feeling during the incident. In the example I provided above, the boy John determined that he was actually feeling afraid, and perhaps a bit jealous.

Fourth, write down the thoughts you had during the incident. Going along with the above example again, John's thoughts may have been things like, "Why do they show my sister more attention?" or "Maybe they like her because she's a girl – or maybe because she is not autistic."

Lastly, identify some objective supporting evidence. Write out some thoughts that would support the things you wrote automatically above. In my example, John may write something like, "The person with the picture was mostly talking about their own child in the photo," or "everyone knows I don't like to have my picture taken anyway. Perhaps this person was just trying to be respectful of my preferences."

Cognitive behavioral therapy can be an effective tool in bringing an autistic person's thoughts into the open and helping them work through those thought processes in a safe and secure way.

# CHAPTER 3: GUIDED IMAGERY

Guided imagery is the practice of mentally walking through a relaxing scene in their minds. The person would first relax as much as possible, then imagine some scene where they would feel calm and relaxed. This would be done in as great detail as possible, involving all the senses. Imagine the scents, the sights, the feeling of what is around you, the sounds you'd be hearing and tastes that you'd associate with that place.

So for example, imagining a relaxing scene on the beach you might note the scent of the saltwater, the sound of crashing waves on the shore and the cries of seagulls in the air, the feel of the sand between your toes and the cool breeze in your hair, the sight of the sun setting behind the pier on the horizon, and the taste of a favorite ice cream or some other treat you might get on a trip to the beach for the day.

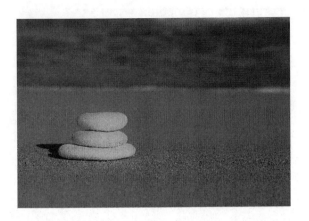

This exercise is good practice for someone on the autism spectrum, as doing this sort of sensory grounding in daily life is a good mind-body exercise throughout the course of their average day.

They may also want to try imagining themselves walking through their school day, replaying a scene during school in which they felt at ease, or meeting a trusted friend or confidante. The point of this exercise is to bring them to a place of safety where they can relax and learn that the feeling of stillness or peace is not a threatening thing.

✽ ✽ ✽

I understand that the two methods for self-soothing mentioned in the previous chapters may not be practical for some with autism – not yet at least. They may only apply to those with high functioning levels, but they do offer hope that something can be done. Studies have proven that early intervention helps children with autism, bringing them closer to a state in which they can communicate their needs and desires, and gain help from the world around them.

The polyvagal theory and its branches of research into the mind and body and how they function together are bringing to light many things we had not previously known. Some of these are showing great promise for the future of how we see autism as a whole, and how we might bring this condition more into the light.

For instance, there is evidence that inflammation alone may have an impact on the symptoms of autism. As the vagus nerve has a direct impact on the inflammation of the gut system, this may be an avenue of research that will provide some great strides. Even now there are reports of changes in diet impacting autistic symptoms, and things like vagus nerve stimulation helping to bring autism into a safer, more manageable place.

# PART FOUR

This last section is going to take us through some physical ailments that are impacted by the tone of the vagus nerve and how we can strengthen the vagus in order to reach our most healthy state. This will include exercises and breathing techniques that anyone may find helpful.

# CHAPTER 1: VAGUS NERVE AND THE BODY

## Healing The Body Through Stimulation Of The Vagus Nerve

Many maladies of the mind and body are affected by the vagus nerve. Its presence is so pervasive among the various systems of the body that it is no wonder such a wide variety of conditions would be touched by this nerve system.

For example, prolonged stress can lead to physical problems such as asthma, colds and flu, cancer, depression, heart disease, stomach ulcers, even eczema and various skin disorders.

We know now that the vagus nerve is responsible for sending the necessary signals to the bodily organs to de-stress, release enzymes and proteins that calm the body and allow relaxation to begin again. However, if the vagus nerve is not doing this signaling effectively, then the long-term effects of stress will continue to rise in the body.

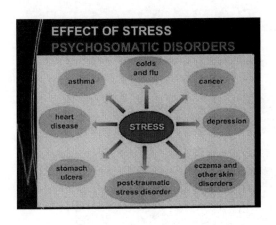

This shows us then how pervasive the effects of stress can be on the body, and just what sort of benefits we can provide ourselves by recognizing the importance of the vagus nerve and its health is on the overall health of the body and mind. Many of the maladies below are chronic illnesses afflicting millions of people in the world. They can be helped to alleviate some of their symptoms by strengthening the vagus nerve as we are going to show.

- Gut health
- Anxiety
- Depression
- Bipolar Disorder
- Attention Deficit Disorder
- Autism
- Epilepsy
- Alzheimer's
- Rheumatoid Arthritis
- Obesity
- Diabetes
- And more…

Next, we will be going through a few of these conditions and detailing how the vagus nerve affects it and how treating it can have an impact on the symptoms.

## Gut Health and Inflammation

Gut health is intrinsically tied to the brain, and the brain to the gut. That may seem odd at first, but when we look at how our neurons actually function, it makes perfect sense.

Neurons, found all throughout our bodies, tell our body how to behave. The vagus nerve, as we have learned, is a major pathway from the gut to the brain and back again. Among other things, stress clogs that pathway, like too much traffic on a freeway in rush hour, and can create gut health issues such as Irritable Bowel Syndrome and Crohn's disease.

Probiotics can help with these afflictions but lowered vagal tone will reduce any effectiveness that these probiotics may have.

Eating foods such as fish like salmon helps tone the vagus nerve, and can help increase your gut health. It is amazing how closely related gut health is to your brain health as well.

Inflammation can and often does begin in the gut. If you are anything like me, I thought that most inflammation was because of torn muscles or overworked strained tendons or ligaments, something more related to the muscular or skeletal structure of the body. While this type of inflammation is certainly a real thing, there is also much that tells us inflammation can be the direct result of bacteria in our gut.

Inflammation can be caused by a heightened presence of cytokines, and studies have shown that stimulating the vagus nerve reduces the level of cytokines in the body.

We speak here of inflammation as it starts in the gut, but it impacts more than just those organs that reside in that part of our abdomen. The inflammation here has a direct impact on the health of the brain, and also is related to many other health issues, including Alzheimer's, anxiety, depression, Rheumatoid arthritis, and in more recent studies, we see that inflammation has an impact on even Autism. There is even a study that was done that showed a correlation between inflammation and aggression caused by the microbiome in our gut being unbalanced.

To promote your best gut health, try foods like salmon, avocados, olive oil, and dark green leafy vegetables. Take care of your gut and your gut will take care of you.

For help in this area, you might try an anti-inflammatory diet. All of these are rich in foods that stimulate the vagus nerve, thus reducing the harmful bacteria that causes inflammation, and increasing those proteins that fight inflammation.

Recipes such as oat porridge, using steel cut or traditional oats, and a generous helping of berries on top for breakfast, or buckwheat porridge. Perhaps some buckwheat pancakes sound good. Scrambled eggs with turmeric could help with inflammation too. Turmeric is potent but is one ingredient well-known to combat inflammation. For dinner perhaps try smoked salmon, avocado, and poached eggs on toast. A pineapple smoothie for dessert will work out wonderful.

These are just some ideas and may not be how you want to eat every day, but something from an anti-inflammatory diet each day could send you on the way to a more healthful state of being.

# Depression

Depression is essentially the opposite of anxiety, with anxiety being based in a fear of the future and depression most usually being based in regret over the past. Yet the vagus nerve has been found to have a profound impact on both conditions. According to a study published in ScienceDaily.com, doctors in China had some very promising results by using a small device just under the skin near the ear to stimulate the vagus nerve in patients suffering from clinical depression. The results showed real improvement with the connection between the neurons and the network in the brain that is usually altered in those suffering from depression.

## Epilepsy

Both epilepsy and depression have been shown to be benefitted by electrical stimulation of the vagus nerve. This should always be done under the supervision of a doctor who understands this method of treatment.

## Obesity and Eating disorders

The vagus nerve has a direct impact on sending neurons from the gut to the stomach and brain regarding the type and frequency of nutrients the gut needs. Basically, a calorie-rich diet tells your vagus nerve that the gut needs this diet. It changes your metabolism, telling your body that more calories are needed, being a possible contributor to overeating. Vagal nerve stimulation has been shown in some studies to prevent weight gain, and in severe cases, a vagal blockade has been used to result in significant weight loss. This block is an implantable device used to stimulate the vagus nerve on the anterior abdominal wall.

The above is the possible way the vagus nerve can have a direct biological impact on our weight gain or weight loss. But the vagus nerve also has an impact on us mentally, psychologically. Another way the vagus nerve can have a direct impact on weight gain is by remembering that the sympathetic and parasympathetic nervous systems are completely focused on the safety of the human body. When the parasympathetic system is trained to receive signals of safety from the process of eating food, it will crave that food more and more.

Remember again that the vagus nerve in its ventral state is all about finding that sense of safety. Children with sensory issues, for example, may actually be seeing food as a danger signal. A child who has a heightened sensitivity to the feel of certain tactile sensations may be associating foods with that feeling, and then be avoiding many foods because of that.

## Diabetes

Recent studies are showing that abdominal vagus nerve stimulation, in particular, helps with the improvement of whole-body glucose uptake, increasing the sensitivity of the body to insulin, which then helped the body reduce glucose in the blood.

✳ ✳ ✳

These are just a few of the issues that stimulating the vagus nerve can help to alleviate. Next, we will discuss some ways to go about stimulating the vagus nerve itself. There are some electronic devices available for this, but we will be discussing the low-cost, natural remedies here. Be sure that whatever method you use, you remember that overstimulating the vagus nerve can cause fainting as it is responsible for lowering the heart rate. Anyone with low blood pressure or heart conditions should proceed with caution and under the direction of a physician.

# CHAPTER 2: TONING YOUR VAGUS

## Toning Exercises

Some damage cannot be healed. There are cases where surgeries have permanently damaged the vagus nerve. Some diseases such as diabetes create damage to the nerve as well, but studies have shown that there is hope in strengthening the vagus nerve that has experienced some forms of tonal loss. Stimulating the vagus nerve is different than flexing a muscle. I see it as more like strumming a piano wire. In keeping it active, the vagus nerve gains myelin where it ought to and remains toned and ready for action where it needs to function the most. These exercises help to tone and strengthen the nerve.

First of all, be aware that stimulating the vagus nerve slows heart rate and respirations. While this is fine when in a state of accelerated heart rate and breathing, you do want to be careful of physically overstimulating the nerve when in a normal, non-panic state. That being said, stimulating the vagus nerve at a reasonable level can help improve many aspects of our physical and mental state.

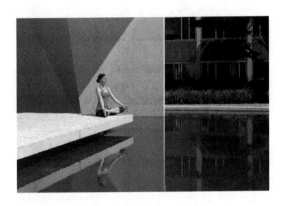

The next section will tell you about some natural and easy methods to keep your vagus nerve in tune with a healthier you.

## Diving Reflex

The diving reflex is a form of breathing that also innervates the vagus nerve. It helps lower your pulse rate and relax your body, so it is actually recommended as an easy trick when facing something daunting, like giving a presentation or going in to a business meeting. Cold water anywhere on your face from your lips to your scalp line will stimulate this reflex. You can also try placing your tongue in cold water or dipping in one finger in cold water.

It is said though that the most effective use of this is when you get your entire face wet and simulate holding your breath as if you were diving into deep water. The reflex works by causing a reaction in the trigeminal nerves, the facial nerves. When these nerves detect water all over the face, they send a message to the vagus nerve to calm the heart. Interestingly, this response only happens in humans when in contact with water.

## Valsalva maneuver

The Valsalva maneuver sounds complicated, but it is really very simple. This is the concept of trying to breathe against a closed airway and is accomplished through taking a breath, then pinching your nose shut and holding your mouth closed while trying to breathe out. Do not be rough on yourself, this one comes with a disclaimer. If you have a heart condition such as coronary heart disease, a congenital heart defect, or other heart conditions, your doctor may advise you not to do it. This maneuver can raise your blood pressure too.

## Connect with others

The first thing that helps tone the vagus nerve is positive social interaction. By flexing the nerve, giving it more signs of positive relationships, we teach the brain how to remap itself. Smiling at a loved one, allowing the shine of love to show in your eyes, the crinkling of the corners of your eyes, bringing up a happy memory and purposely smiling at it. Smile more, smile with your eyes, allow your face to show happiness.

Allow yourself to enter into connection with other people. Practice intentional listening, practice caring about others. Amazingly this will improve both your social engagement system as well as theirs.

## Be vocal

Sing loud and sing proud. There is no reason to hold back at this point. The very act of singing alone helps to stimulate the nerve, as it lies just behind the jawline and is connected to the tongue as well. Listening to music is great but singing along with it will improve your vagus nerve tone. You do not have to sing well, just sing. Even humming or chanting will work this way. So grab a mic, go do karaoke in your living room. Hum your favorite tune while driving down the road.

Polyvagal research has also shown that music tunes the vagus nerve itself. Participation in that music uses the cranial muscles and translates calm and safety to the vagus nerve, soothing the heart and helping it work better. Music literally adds health to your body.

## Gargle

Gargling also works to stimulate the vocal cords in the same way as singing or humming, and this also helps to tone the vagus nerve as well.

## Cold Exposure

Exposure to cold is an easy way to tone your vagus nerve, so splashing the face with cold water, or creating a cold sensation, especially on the forehead and chest. You can also rinse your hands or feet in cold water or take a cold bath or shower.

## Simple Massage

Another way is by massaging the neck along the carotid sinus. A simple pressure massage can help stimulate the vagus nerve. Seizures can be reduced through a neck massage, and a foot massage can help keep your blood pressure and heart rate low.

## Relax

Simply relaxing helps stimulate the vagus nerve as well. Sit quietly and allow all your muscles to relax. Let your face go slack, your neck, shoulders, arms, and legs. Then slowly smile and release your breath in a long slow exhale.

I know of one family who tried what they called "hug therapy." The mother and daughter were having a difficult time connecting over a few things, and so during this time, the mother would pull her daughter in for a hug and hold her until they both felt relaxed in the hug. As soon as the relaxation happened, they released the hug and smiled. The mother was comfortable with this before the daughter was, but very soon the daughter also became comfortable and their connection deepened. They were able to be present for each other on a more meaningful level.

## Diet

Lastly, a better diet is also one method of stimulating the vagus nerve. Try eating bitter foods to stimulate vagal nerve receptor sites, such as coffee, green tea, cranberries, citrus peel, or dandelion greens. Bitter foods, in particular, create a response that wakes up the vagus nerve.

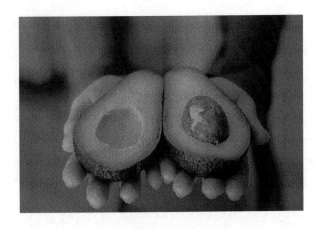

## Intermittent Fasting

Another method in the area of diet is something that is not actually a dietary change. Intermittent fasting is becoming more popular lately, as it is not a change in *what* you eat but is a change in *when* you eat. This method of eating is often used in an attempt to slim down, lose bad fat while retaining the good. The pattern of when you eat is what stimulates the vagus nerve. It is said that the body absorbs fat best when in the fasting state, which occurs eight to twelve hours after the last meal. This means the intermittent fasting pattern can follow different models.

A popular pattern to follow is the Leangains model, which is sixteen hours of fasting followed by eight hours of eating. Eat within that window only, then fast for the sixteen. Women may find it more beneficial to change this a little, eating during a ten-hour window, and fasting for fourteen hours. It is that simple.

You might also try the intermittent fasting one or two days a week, or every other day rather than starting right off with the new pattern every day of the week. Fortunately, this method is not hard to learn. You most likely already are in the habit of eating at the same time every day without even thinking about it. It is not hard to change this pattern to a daily method of only eating within a certain time period.

In this model, you may skip breakfast or lunch, you may only eat twice during that eight or ten-hour window. You might need to eat slightly bigger meals or be more mindful of how many calories you are taking in during the week. Being mindful of what your body needs is a good thing. So try this if you'd like to work on toning your vagus nerve and lose some weight at the same time.

## Pressure Points

In the center of the underside of your arm, three finger widths from the base of the palm there is a pressure point between the two tendons of your forearm. This is said to be an acupuncture pressure point that will reach the vagus nerve. Applying pressure here is said to help with stress, anxiety, heart palpitations, and even nausea from motion sickness and pregnancy.

This should not create discomfort, so if it does, lighten your pressure.

## Exercise

Studies have shown that just five minutes of aerobic exercise can begin to reduce stress. These studies have also shown that exercising in the morning will enhance your parasympathetic system, while exercising in the evening will activate the sympathetic system. This means that you will sleep better at night if you exercise in the morning than if you exercise at night. This makes a lot of sense if you look at exercise as telling your brain that your need for energy is high for the next few hours. It will keep your body attuned and ready to go for several hours after the exercise session has ended.

* * *

Lastly, we will be looking at some breathing techniques that can help you keep your vagus nerve in good shape and propel you along the path of good health and wellbeing.

# CHAPTER 3: BETTER BREATHING

## Techniques

Breathing in a calm relaxed way can be a very effective way to regain control and tone your vagus nerve to help keep you in that safe and social state. A couple of things to remember - inhaling is a function of the sympathetic nervous system, that portion that tells us to either fight or flee when danger is present. The exhale is the part of breathing that is linked to the parasympathetic nervous system. Even in the act of breathing these two systems work together each and every time. Because of this, breathing exercises are like tensing and relaxing a muscle. Taking too many deep breaths in too short of a time can cause you to hyperventilate, so please be aware and watch your breathing. Stop if you begin to feel dizzy.

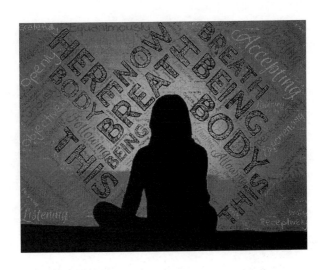

There are different types of breathing exercises you can try. Mixing and matching for your own personal needs will be best, but here are some examples of a few and in what situations some of them might be best to try.

## Lengthening Your Exhale

First, you can try to lengthen your exhale. Before taking a deep breath, exhale everything in your lungs then let your lungs inflate back up again naturally. You can then try to exhale a little longer than you inhaled, such as inhaling to a count of four and exhaling to a count of six. This can be practiced anywhere from two to five minutes.

## Diaphragmatic Breathing

Intentional, diaphragmatic breathing exercises the vagus nerve. These should be done when already in a calm, quiet state. Lie on your back with your knees slightly bent and your head on a pillow. You may also like to place a pillow under your knees for further comfort.

You will want to feel your diaphragm moving, so place one hand on your upper chest, and the other just below your rib cage. After this, inhale slowly through your nose. You will feel your stomach up to your hand. While doing this, try not to move your other hand at all.

When you exhale, purse your lips together and tighten your stomach muscles, keeping the hand on your chest perfectly still.

Later you may want to place a book on your chest for an added challenge. Once you have mastered belly breathing while lying down, you might want to increase the challenge by sitting up, and then later on, perhaps you can practice this type of breathing while doing your daily activities.

## Alternate Nostril Breathing

Next is alternate nostril breathing, another breathing practice used for relaxation. This breathing technique helps to improve cardiovascular function and to lower heart rate, all by improving the vagus nerve's tone. This is a more strenuous technique, so it is best to practice on an empty stomach and when you are feeling neither sick nor congested

First, seat yourself comfortably. Then slowly raise your right hand and gently close your right nostril.

Lift up your right hand toward your nose, bending your first and middle fingers down toward your palm. Leave your other fingers extended.

Exhale, remembering to keep your breath smooth and even throughout this exercise, then use your right thumb to close your right nostril. At this point, you will inhale through your left nostril, then immediately and gently close your left nostril with your right hand's pinky and ring finger. Allow your thumb to lift, letting yourself breathe out through your right nostril. Then inhale through the right and close the nostril again. Open your left nostril again, exhaling through that side.

This is one cycle. Continue this breathing pattern for up to five minutes, finishing your session with an exhale on the left side.

## Pursed Lip Breathing

This one is much simpler. Pursed lip breathing can be practiced at any time throughout the day but may be most useful during times of slightly strenuous activity – climbing stairs, bending, or lifting small items. This is done by relaxing your shoulders, then breathing in slowly through your nose, keeping your mouth closed. Breathe in for a count of two, then purse your lips together as if you are getting ready to whistle. Now you exhale through your pursed lips for a count of four.

## Four-Count Pattern Breathing

For the next breathing exercise, you will sit with one hand on your chest, the other on your stomach. Breathe in slowly, letting the breath fill your lungs as you breathe in through your nose. Hold your breath for four seconds, then breathe out slowly until all the air is out. Repeat this process four more times.

## Coherent Breathing

Then there is resonant or coherent breathing. The goal here is breathing five full breaths for each minute. To attain this goal, you simply breathe in for a count of five and then breathe out for a count of five. Continue the pattern for a few minutes.

Remember that constant chest breathing leaves your sympathetic nervous system closer to activation. The deeper, abdominal breathing tells the brain that we are in a safe place, and triggers that vagus nerve to send its signals of calm to the brain and the rest of the body.

# CONCLUSION

In this book we've explored the vagus nerve, searched for ways to enter into real healing, and learned about the true need for connection that all humans have.

When we create safety for ourselves, our body and mind can work together as they were designed to do. I have found that safety is essential for creativity, for connection, for thriving. It is also interesting to note that creativity and connection to other people provide us with safety.

An experienced horse rider will pay attention when his horse stops short, ears pricked forward and staring into the forest. Or when the horse shies from a spot in the trail, insisting on going around a suspicious patch of bushes instead of through it. The wise rider will pay attention, knowing that the horse can sense some things that he as a human cannot. Just as a rider listens to the cues his horse gives, we would be foolish to ignore the cues that our body gives us as it senses our environment.

Our body is the vehicle given to us to get us through this life. It senses things that our conscious brain cannot always understand quickly, and its reactions need to be taken into account when making decisions.

Going forward, I hope you will be able to use the techniques learned here to live your best life and help others to live their best life as well.

# QUESTIONS FOR FURTHER STUDY

### 1. Does the Polyvagal Theory cure PTSD?

The Polyvagal Theory is a model for approaching therapy. Its effectiveness will vary from individual to individual. This is true of every model of therapy, no matter its basis or theoretical model. No one can promise anyone a definite cure. All anyone can do is offer a way to move forward on the journey to health. The safe and social model does seem to resonate with many people suffering from PTSD and other traumas.

### 2. Will the methods for stimulating the vagus nerve cure me?

The stimulation of the vagus nerve acts as an aid to improving your health in specific areas. It impacts your internal organs in ways we are still learning about.

### 3. Is the Polyvagal Theory the only model for therapy?

No, there are other models that therapists use throughout the field. The Polyvagal Theory itself forms the foundation for a multitude of therapeutic directions. It is not necessarily just one succinct thought process, but rather a basis for determining how to help people begin their journey to overcoming trauma and neurologically affected syndromes.

### 4. How do other models of therapy fit in with the Polyvagal Theory?

Since the Polyvagal Theory is a building block, a place to start, it can and does fit in quite nicely with many other models for therapy. It does not have to overwhelm these other models. It can and does blend in with them, creating the needed plan for each individual as they find it useful and show progress on their own unique journey.

### 5. Is the Polyvagal Theory meant to be a cure-all for all illnesses?

Not a cure-all, no. Within the Polyvagal Theory lies the notion that many ailments can show improvement through a more natural, holistic method of caring for both the body and the mind. By using the body's natural neurological responses, we can use the processes already in place to further healing in a multitude of ways.

# REFERENCES

Autism Facts and Figures. (2018). Retrieved from https://www.autismspeaks.org/autism-facts-and-figures.

Bergland, C. (2016, July 6). Vagus Nerve Stimulation Dramatically Reduces Inflammation. Retrieved from https://www.psychologytoday.com/us/blog/the-athletes-way/201607/vagus-nerve-stimulation-dramatically-reduces-inflammation.

Bergland, C. (n.d.). Face-to-Face Connectedness, Oxytocin, and Your Vagus Nerve. Retrieved May 19, 2017, from https://www.psychologytoday.com/us/blog/the-athletes-way/201705/face-face-connectedness-oxytocin-and-your-vagus-nerve.

Elsevier. (2016, February 4). New non-invasive form of vagus nerve stimulation works to treat depression. Retrieved from https://www.sciencedaily.com/releases/2016/02/160204111728.htm.

Gill, L. (2017, November 25). Understanding and Working with the Window of Tolerance. Retrieved from https://www.attachment-and-trauma-treatment-centre-for-healing.com/blogs/understanding-and-working-with-the-window-of-tolerance.

Godfrey, N., Weidemeier, U., Cappello, T., Labe, D., Hyde, M., Susan, … Sarra, K. (2018, April 13). Polyvagal Theory and How Trauma Impacts the Body. Retrieved from https://www.nicabm.com/trauma-polyvagal-theory-and-how-trauma-impacts-the-body/.

Hall, B. (2019, March 21). What Counts as Play? 5 Criteria of the Most Vital Activity for Kids. Retrieved from https://www.stack.com/a/what-counts-as-play-5-criteria-of-the-most-vital-activity-for-kids.

Headley, B., Koch, L., Johansen, M., Buczynski, R., Leyton, E., & Stoeva, E. (2018, April 4). The Polyvagal Theory in Action – How Heart Rate Figures into Trauma Treatments. Retrieved from https://www.nicabm.com/the-polyvagal-theory-in-action-how-heart-rate-figures-into-trauma-treatments/.

Howes, R., & Porges, S. (n.d.). Wearing Your Heart on Your Face: The Polyvagal Circuit in the Consulting Room. Retrieved from https://www.pesi.com/blog/details/967/wearing-your-heart-on-your-face-the-polyvagal-circuit.

Keown, A. (2019, July 11). New Insights into the Vagus Nerve Could Change the Way Diabetes is Treated. Retrieved October 15, 2019, from https://www.biospace.com/article/new-insights-into-the-vagus-nerve-could-change-the-way-diabetes-is-treated

Pietrangelo, A. (2018, July 2). How to Recognize the Signs of Mental and Emotional Abuse. Retrieved from https://www.healthline.com/health/signs-of-mental-abuse.

Ropp, T. (2017, September 5). 12 Ways to Unlock the Powers of the Vagus Nerve. Retrieved from https://upliftconnect.com/12-ways-unlock-powers-vagus-nerve/.

Rosenfeld, J. (2018, November 13). 9 Fascinating Facts About the Vagus Nerve. Retrieved from http://mentalfloss.com/article/65710/9-nervy-facts-about-vagus-nerve.

Schäfer, T., Huron, D., Shanahan, D., & Sedlmeier, P. (2015, August 5). The sounds of safety: stress and danger in music perception. Retrieved from https://www.ncbi.nlm.nih.gov/pmc/articles/PMC4524892/.

Seltzer, L. F. (2015, July 8). Trauma and the Freeze Response: Good, Bad, or Both. Retrieved from https://www.psychologytoday.com/us/blog/evolution-the-self/201507/trauma-and-the-freeze-response-good-bad-or-both

Siniscalco, D., Schultz, S., Brigida, A. L., & Antonucci, N. (2018, June 4). Inflammation and Neuro-Immune Dysregulations in Autism Spectrum Disorders. Retrieved from https://www.ncbi.nlm.nih.gov/pmc/articles/PMC6027314/.

Made in the USA
San Bernardino, CA
23 November 2019